Rebuilding Your life After a Gray Divorce

A Path to Healing, Significance, and Joy

Pat Fenner

Author and Podcast Producer Pat Fenner has designed a compelling and inspiring framework to create a life of peace and productivity after a gray divorce.

Table Of Contents

ACKNOWLEDGEMENTS 1
INTRODUCTION: MY STORY 2
PART 1: THE STRENGTHS FRAMEWORK 12
   1. S: Embrace Simplicity 13
   2. T: Take Care of Yourself 18
   3. R: Rebuild Trust 28
   4. E: Expect the Best 35
   5. N: Know Your Boundaries 40
   6. G: Be Gentle with Yourself 47
   7. T: Be Thankful 54
   8. H: Have a Sense of Humor 59
   9. S: Show Forgiveness 63
PART 2: MOVING FORWARD WITH STRENGTH 69
   10. Suddenly Supporting Yourself 70
   11. Divorce and Your Adult Children 74
   12. On Brokenness 78
   13. Holidays and Happiness 83
   14. Quick Wins 88
   15. Final Thoughts 98
   16. Recommended Resources 100
   17. Notes 102

ACKNOWLEDGEMENTS

There are so many who have made it possible for this book to see the light of day, and who enabled me to see any light as I moved through a dark tunnel. First of all, to Jesus, Who is the reason I *don't* believe in coincidences, and is always at work in my life, whether or not I see it. My adult kiddos, who supported me and encouraged me to accomplish what I couldn't see happening, until it finally started happening. I owe a true debt of gratitude to my sister, Cathi, too, for being a constant cheerleader and never-ending source of support.

Friends from years ago, Ginny, Candy, and Ruthie - wise women and prayer warriors who lifted me in prayer even - or especially - when I wasn't able to. My dear friend Tracey, who God truly dropped into my life when we both needed each other, and who continues to make me laugh, think, and pray.

The counseling and coaching so gently delivered by Virginia, Michelle, and Amy - who never stopped encouraging me to explore and accept who God made me to be, and encouraged me to move forward in my gifts and strengths.

I'm also grateful for my amazing editor Lois, without whose help, this would have stayed a jumbled mess. And, last but certainly not least, graphics-pro, Phil, who so patiently designed (and *re*designed) the cover.

If this book helps even one soul on this journey, I will be satisfied that it was all worth it, and grateful that God saw fit to use my story to build up another.

INTRODUCTION: MY STORY

"The past is a place of reference, not a place of residence."
~ Roy T. Bennet

"You don't 'get over' divorce, you heal from it."
~ Julia F.

I didn't plan to write this book. At first, I didn't even *want* to write it.

For too long, I tried to hide the story I'm about to tell you. I believed it reflected a huge personal failure—that *I* was a failure, and it would be best if I simply packed away the whole event and moved on. The conversations I had—with my ex-husband, with counselors, with myself—were often pointed and painful. I felt raw on every level and isolated from anyone who might have a scant notion of what I was going through. I was ashamed of an entire chunk of my life.

Why? Because I'm a Christian. I believe in marriage for life. *And* I'm divorced.

It was hard for me to write that last sentence. Even now—years after my marriage officially ended—it's still a bit difficult for me to read.

Growing up, I was taught marriage was for life or until the death of a spouse. I don't remember one relative of mine who was divorced. In fact, I didn't know *anyone* who was divorced until I went to college. When I met the man who became my husband, his birth parents were divorced. By the time of their deaths, they'd each been married three times. (For the sake of their two sons, however, they remained congenial over the years, a unique arrangement that occasionally created some awkward situations.)

Several years after we got married, we moved to the Bible Belt where the "marriage-for-life" mindset was the norm. We had kids by then, and most, if not all, of our friends were married. Even so, I sometimes encountered relationships that left me feeling unsettled, as if something was slightly off, but I couldn't quite put my finger on what it was. Of course, we *never* talked about it. If anything was wrong at home, it was supposed to be a matter of prayer and end there. We may not have been told we would "go to hell" if we divorced our spouses, but the implication was there, and thus, the fear of it.

Sadly, as I rediscover friends from that time of my life on social media, I can count eight couples I was fairly close to who have since divorced. I had my suspicions about a few of them, but I never knew for sure that they were experiencing marital pain. I guess we were supposed to suffer in silence.

I tell you all that to say this: For me to get where I am today was truly a journey. It was mostly lonely, sometimes a slog, often riddled with self-reproach and negative feelings. But while the process of researching and writing about this chapter of my life has provided an extra dose of personal therapy, this book isn't for me. It's for you ...

- If you are newly divorced and unsure how to navigate a life that looms dismal and daunting before you.

- If you've been divorced for a while and feel stuck in bitterness, regret, or sadness.
- In either case, if you feel as if you're spinning your wheels and getting nowhere, or you're frozen with fear and unable to move on.
- If you're feeling isolated within a community of faith that doesn't support your struggle and suffering as a divorced woman.
- If you feel like a failure because of where life has brought you.

If you see yourself on that list, I'm praying the strategies that helped me move from a place of turmoil and tears to one of peace and joy will do the same for you.

Specifically, gray divorce is defined as divorce past the age of fifty, and often after a marriage of ten or more years. The parameters are important to note, because divorce after this age creates unique circumstances, and women in this demographic share many common characteristics. While some didn't attend college, others graduated but left the workforce shortly after marriage and then spent years at home, raising children. Although we may be good at running a house on a budget, many of us were not actively involved in the bigger-picture aspects of finances, such as making larger purchases (cars, homes, etc.), handling investments, insurance, wills and legacy planning. This lack of financial experience may not sound like a big deal, but in this season of life, it can become one.

As of this writing, the divorce rate of Americans over fifty has doubled since 1990, and *tripled* for those past sixty-five.[1] While gray divorce puts women at a high financial risk, there are also emotional, psychological, and health-related consequences.[2] In a perfect world, few would consider divorce the best option. As one financial advisor noted, "Maybe the money would be better spent on marital counseling than on a divorce attorney."[3]

If you're reading this book, however, that ship has already sailed.

The papers have been signed and filed. The joint accounts have been canceled. The property and assets you owned together have been divvied up. It's time to move on.

And so, my friend, we shall.

Let me share a sobering story to explain why this is so important.

Shortly after I moved into my current home, I met a woman at a local business networking meeting. We seemed to have a lot in common and decided to have lunch together to continue an interesting conversation we'd started after the meeting. Over a steaming bowl of fresh ramen, we talked about our lives and lessons learned. At some point, she shared she was divorced, too, but it wasn't clear to me for how long. After we asked for the check, I casually asked her when she'd gotten divorced. Her answer broke my heart.

Her divorce was finalized *fifteen years ago*.

For fifteen years, she had been living with periodic bouts of depression so severe she required regular medication. For fifteen years, she had been struggling with bitterness and resentment that colored her perception of relationships in general and made it difficult for her to make friends. For fifteen years, she had been hesitant to travel, try new things, develop personal interests and skills, and meet new people. She admitted she felt her world was slowly closing in on her as the years passed.

I don't want that for you, and I suspect you don't want it either. Happily, it doesn't have to be that way.

Divorce, as painful and crushing as it may be, can open the door to countless opportunities. I'm not saying it's the only way to access these opportunities. And I'm certainly not suggesting it's a preferred method. But I *am* saying that divorce won't keep you from living a full life, one you may never have dreamed possible.

When I was newly married, I would hear about couples splitting after thirty or forty years of marriage and think, *How could anyone live together that long and then break up? Couldn't they just "suck it up" after that much time?* (I know—ouch!) While my ex's parents were divorced, we had always said we might kill each other, but we'd never divorce (which was supposed to be funny, I guess).

I have no desire to discredit my ex or paint him as the bad guy. I know full well that it takes two to tango and there are two sides to every failed marriage story. I also know that despite prayer, counseling, and talking things over (or *not* talking them over), something happened to both of us over the years. Eventually, that "something" developed into a chasm that led to brokenness too painful to live with. (And, ironically, just as painful to learn to live without.)

When we finally divorced in 2023, we had been married for thirty-seven years. We had five children ranging in age from eighteen to thirty-four. I'll add other bits of information along the way to provide context, but for the most part, I'll spare you further details. I'm not looking for pity, for one thing, but I also don't want to share anything that might distract or trigger you in your situation. Rather than rile up your emotions as you read, I want to help you work and grow through your own story. As I said before, what I *will* share are the strategies that helped me work through the most painful period of my life—a time when I questioned my self-worth, my abilities, my past, my future, and my faith.

I'm not exaggerating. Divorce hit me to the core, and it totally broke me. The good news is that I'm still alive. And because of that, I know my story isn't over.

I'm still on the journey. I still have days when I feel swallowed up by despair and depression, along with many other days when life feels like sunshine and lollipops. On *all* those days, however, I know this truth: God is good, and He loves me. That knowledge—that firm conviction—gets me through the bad days and makes the good days even better.

If you're reading these words, my heart breaks for you. I know you may be in a place you don't want to be. You may find yourself alone and lonely, struggling to make sense of where you are and where you're going. It may not bring you much comfort right now, but please remember that I'm praying for you. Whether or not you're a believer, you can absolutely trust that everything happens for a reason. And even if that reason remains elusive, by the time you get to the end of this short book, I fervently hope that you'll see a way to move on.

I've used the acronym STRENGTHS as the framework for this book because strength was what I prayed for most in the early days of my divorce. I worked hard to be present for my adult kids and my clients, but inside I felt like I was stuck at the bottom of a deep well. *Courage* was my Word of the Year during that season, and it definitely helped me to forge ahead. But strength was what I needed to get through each day, and it became a crucial craving.

The strategies I've outlined are not listed in any particular order; they are presented in a way that fits the acronym. They all work together, and you may decide to pick and choose the order in which you approach them. It's your journey, and you get to travel it any way that works for you.

That said, I encourage you to take your time reading this book. Move through one chapter or section at a time, at your own pace. Jot down notes or thoughts or personal applications on the journal pages. Be mindful and intentional about your healing and growth, and remind yourself—as often as you need to and in whatever way works best—that the only contest that matters is achieving your own personal best.

I recently became an *abuela* (grandmother) for the third time, and something about watching this newborn bundle of joy has hit an unexpected chord in me. Baby M is learning so much. At times he cries for no apparent reason. When he looks around, his eyes seem to cross as he adjusts to his growing abilities and depth perception. Soon he'll be crawling and exploring. Before we know it, he'll be running around and getting into shenanigans.

But he needs to develop a great deal of strength and many skills before he gets to that point.

Boy, do I identify with this phase of growth as I think about my post-divorce recovery—

everything from the spontaneous tears to needing to build strength in different areas of life. My perception is constantly adjusting; even now, I remain in exploratory mode. And I'll probably have my own shenanigans along the way too. Beyond that, I've had the privilege of watching five children go through all those steps as they become the capable, talented, and unique creations of God that they are. That's a good deal of experience watching people grow, change, and blossom. I'm going to claim that potential for myself, and I encourage you to do the same.

In fact, let's both take a moment and say the following out loud: *I look forward to blooming into the capable, talented, and unique creation of God that I am!*

If you don't believe it now, that's fine. Someday you will.

Before we move on, I want to share one more thing: I don't believe in coincidences.

When I was going through my divorce and rebuilding a life afterward, so many things happened that could have been chalked up to coincidence. Events I attended, people I met, movies I saw, podcasts I listened to, and clients or opportunities that came my way, all of which had an indelible effect on my life and came about when I was ready and needed them most. I've included some of these experiences in this story, and I will forever think of them as the coincidences I *don't* believe in. As you work toward health and wholeness, I hope you'll begin to see the people and opportunities that fall into your life at just the right time as more than just coincidence too.

No matter what you're going through, isn't it comforting and somehow empowering to know that Somebody smarter and stronger than you has your back?

YOUR TURN
At the end of each chapter, you'll find a lined page for your own thoughts. So why not start now? What are you thinking about, feeling, or hoping to learn as you get ready to rebuild *your* life?

PART 1
THE STRENGTHS FRAMEWORK

1.
S: Embrace Simplicity

"Simplicity is the essence of happiness."
~ Cedric Bledsoe

"If your mind isn't clouded by unnecessary things, then this is the best season of your life."
~ Wu-Men

The two years prior to my divorce will forever be a blur. So much was happening. Having to work through the emotional and logistical fallout from the Covid-19 pandemic at the same time made everything more stressful and intense.

My father-in-law died in 2020 and my mother-in-law the year after. We lost them both in less than twelve months and were finally arranging to inter them up north. Wrapping up their estates ensured an active and long to-do list. We had one child who had just graduated from college and was trying to figure out next steps in a world that seemed to have more closed doors than open (literally and figuratively). And another, preparing for college, was overwhelmed with the whole process. Sadly, I wasn't in a great position to support or be there for either of them.

Logistically, my then-husband and I needed to have some conversations about moving forward. Divorce was part of those conversations, but nothing was in motion yet. Work kept him on the road most of the time, so I was trying to imagine how I was going to manage living alone in a four-bedroom house, three hours away from my grown children—the people who meant the most to me in the world. If I decided to move, how and where would that happen? With divorce on the horizon, I began looking into my housing options. I discovered that, with no employment history and no full-time job, it would be difficult—if not impossible—to buy or even rent a home or apartment. While I had already started a "side gig" and was making some money, I learned I'd need at least two years of tax returns to even *apply* for a mortgage or a rental.

I felt stuck between a rock and a hard place.

Other financial questions plagued me too:

- How would I support myself?
- Who would hire a middle-aged woman who hadn't been employed in more than thirty years?
- How do I find—and pay for—a lawyer and protect my future?

But even worse were the emotional/psychological/spiritual questions:

- What was my extended family going to think?
- What were my (mostly conservative) friends going to think?
- What does God make of all this?
- Should I have tried harder?
- *Was it really so horrible being married to me?*

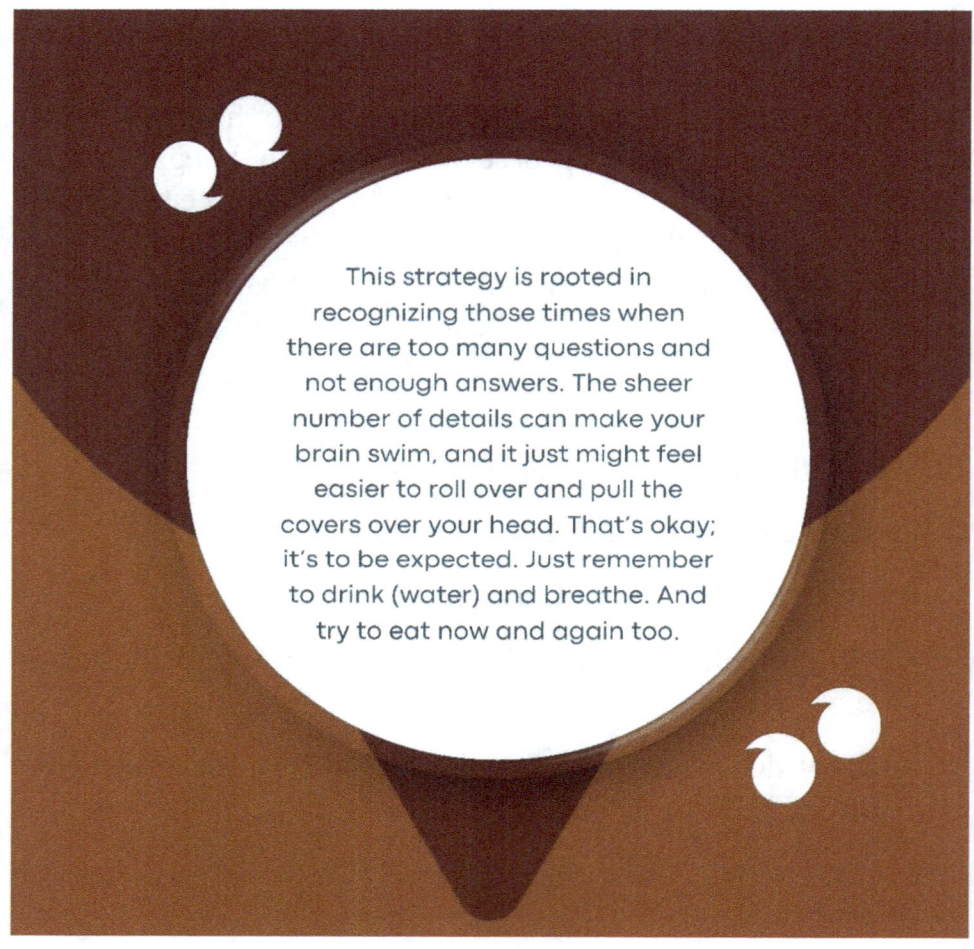

This strategy is rooted in recognizing those times when there are too many questions and not enough answers. The sheer number of details can make your brain swim, and it just might feel easier to roll over and pull the covers over your head. That's okay; it's to be expected. Just remember to drink (water) and breathe. And try to eat now and again too.

If you're anything like me, you may find yourself replaying worst-case scenarios in your mind. Thinking—or worse yet, *overthinking*—your next step. Your next five steps. Your next twenty-five steps. Feeling powerless tends to lead us down dark, dead-end alleys. As my wise daughter reminds me, "It's so easy to spend too much of our lives worrying about things that never happen."

We create the ideal environment for powerlessness when we overthink things or attempt to imagine those next twenty-five steps. Trying to cover all our bases or create the ultimate to-do list provides ample opportunities for our minds to become overwhelmed and start a cycle of negative self-talk. That cycle is easy to get into but uber-hard to get out of—even in an ideal world, there is only so much we can think and do and plan for at one time.

All we really need to do is to take the next step. (Please notice, that's *singular*.)

You may feel you have no choice about simplicity at first. Some days, just getting out of bed and dressed may feel like an Olympic event. On other days, you may feel a burst of energy and do a load of laundry (I'm only half-joking). There's no pattern, no way to predict the good and bad days, and certainly no distinct roadmap.

Embracing simplicity is an overarching concept to keep in mind as you read this book. Take each day as it comes. Try one strategy (or simply tweak one) until it comes naturally, and only if you find it helpful. Overcomplicating things is bound to lead you to some unnecessary places, often back in bed with the covers pulled over your head. Do yourself a favor and be your own best friend right now.

Keep it simple, sweetheart.

YOUR TURN:
How will you begin to embrace simplicity in your life?

2.
T: TAKE CARE OF YOURSELF

"In the event of an emergency, put your own oxygen mask on first." ~ every flight attendant on every airline

"You cannot serve from an empty vessel." ~ Eleanor Brownn

For most of my life, I was so used to doing things for other people I never gave much time, attention, or effort to taking care of myself. I don't say that to brag or come across as a martyr.

It's just a statement of fact. So when I found myself alone after all those years, the first thing I had to learn was how to take care of myself—in many different ways.

Health

Step one was to find a doctor and get a physical. I had arranged or scheduled annual checkups and medical appointments for the kids over the years, but I often didn't have the time or money to do the same for myself. I realized I needed to lose some weight and make a few other changes to ensure better health for myself.

It felt kind of strange, honestly. It almost seemed selfish to take care of myself. But then it occurred to me that I had been pouring out of an empty pitcher for many years. Now I no longer had any excuses. I was alone and only responsible for myself. And there was no good reason to not take care of me. This is the easiest area to get started in self-care—just make the darn appointments! If you must, pretend you're doing it for one of your kids or "asking for a friend."

Finances

Shortly after my divorce, I realized I needed to get my financial house in order. I was not alone: I learned this can be a huge challenge for many women in their fifties and sixties. And the more I learned, the more compelled I felt to do something that would help others. So besides getting a handle on my finances, including managing investments and preparing for retirement, I began working toward becoming a licensed financial advisor. The process quickly went from needing to help myself to wanting to help others. I'm not suggesting this path for everyone. But I strongly encourage you to learn what you need to know to make informed choices. It's *your* money, and now *your* future. Check out Chapter 10 for a deeper discussion of this critical topic.

Emotions

When I began taking self-care seriously, it was apparent to me that I would need the help of a professional counselor. I was still grieving the loss of both my in-laws whom I had cared for—and cared about—for many years. Four of my five children had left home, and there was grief in the transition to an empty nest. Our younger daughter was a college freshman, still trying to decide what to do with her life. On top of all that, there was the grief of losing a marriage. The realization that my circumstances were changing in a big way was foundationally motivating. (In Chapter 3, you'll discover how counseling can help in ways that go beyond emotional healing.)

You'll also need to start establishing boundaries around your emotions. It's important to note that boundaries are *not* tools to regulate others' behavior, but rather deciding how you will respond to that behavior. For example, if someone insists on talking about your ex and you find it painful, you can establish a boundary by telling them if they continue to do that, you'll leave the room. If they keep it up, simply follow through without drama or rancor. Don't allow your emotions to be dragged through the mud. (See Chapter 5 for a more thorough discussion of boundaries.)

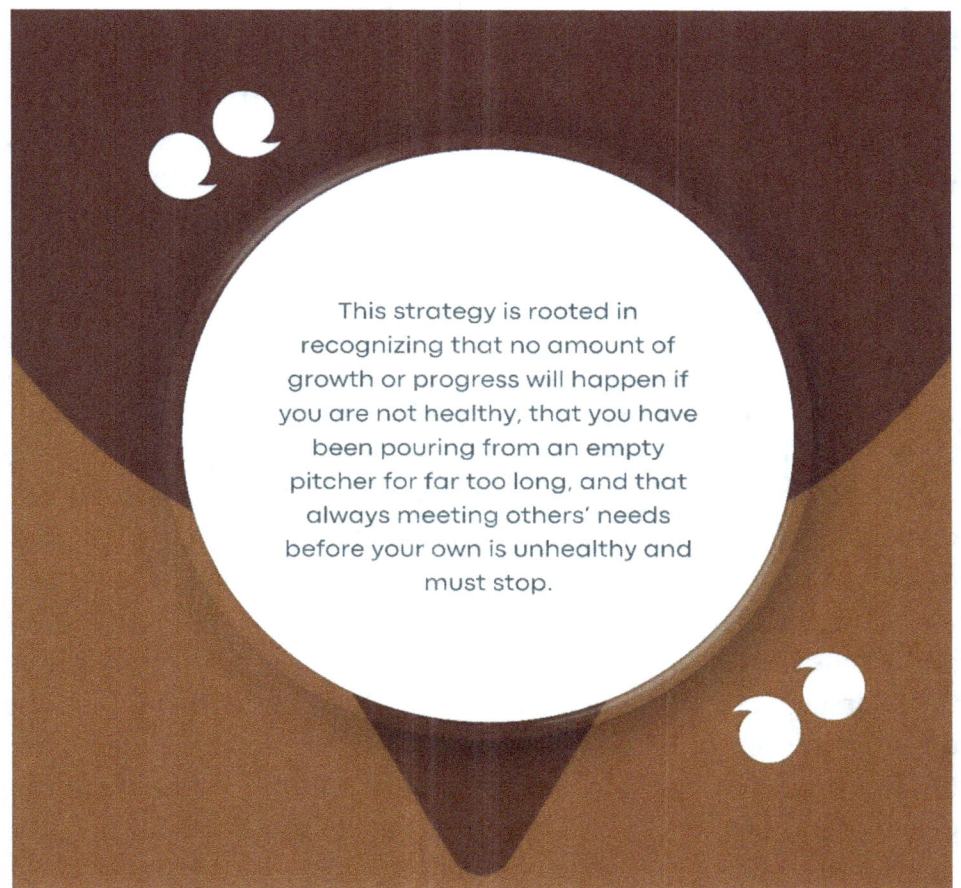

This strategy is rooted in recognizing that no amount of growth or progress will happen if you are not healthy, that you have been pouring from an empty pitcher for far too long, and that always meeting others' needs before your own is unhealthy and must stop.

Dealing with loneliness is another aspect of emotional self-care. The first time you go to a movie, a museum, or out to eat by yourself may be awkward, especially if you're a social person. But it's important to know the distinction between being *alone* and being *lonely*. Initially, it's easy to get lost in a pity party and feel alone in the world, and I'm not suggesting you ignore or suppress that emotion. But please, please, *please* don't stay there! Learn to feel comfortable with your own company. Explore your thoughts and feelings. Enjoy your internal observations and conversation. Engage with memories—the happy ones and those of overcoming adversities. Don't rush into dating because you "need" to have someone else in your life. Learn to be strong on your own so you can have healthier relationships if and/or when you are ready for another special someone down the road. Being open to change enables you to better embrace new opportunities—and people—as they present themselves.

Faith

My faith was one of the biggest areas of my life that took a hit just before my divorce and for a while thereafter. At the same time, it's also what got me through the darkest nights and the most challenging days. There were times when I would rail against God and wonder why He was allowing this to happen, questioning where He'd gone and why He'd left me. Other times, I prayed for clarity and help in whatever form He would offer and whatever way I could receive. I was scared that by failing at my marriage, I was somehow failing God. I would spend some days crying out to Him, or just crying. Other days I felt so close to Him it was almost like He was gently holding me in His arms. On those mornings, I'd drink my coffee at the kitchen table overlooking our green, lush backyard and talk to Him as if He were physically sitting there with me. (I have to admit, talking out loud to an invisible God sometimes made me think I was losing it.) Mostly, though, I felt like I was letting Him down.

Looking back, I see He was there the whole time, walking with me through the valley. Just like I would sometimes have to stand by and watch our children have temper tantrums out of frustration when they were little, God was there watching me as I worked through it all. He brought the right counselors as I needed them, along with friends who would stick by me, sit and listen, and pray for me. He facilitated circumstances I couldn't orchestrate myself. The kind of help He knew I needed, He provided in his perfect timing. I'm not saying He arranged for my divorce to happen just so I would have a stronger faith. But much like an addict sometimes needs to hit bottom before he or she gets better, I needed to hit bottom to comprehend exactly how much I needed God— how much I depended on Him and how critical it was to have daily communion with Him in my life.

If you're a person of faith, let me encourage you that no matter how bleak the days are, stay the course and dig deep. Get Christian counseling. Find a good church, one that supports, nourishes, and challenges you. Spend time in prayer every day, even if it's "just" conversational prayer. In fact, I'd go so far as to suggest that you maintain a running conversation with God. Time with Him is the ultimate safe space, and it is only through Him that healing comes.

Intellect

This is a great time to ignite—or reignite, as the case may be—a lifestyle of learning. If you hated school and didn't feel like you were a great student, it may have been because the traditional, classroom mode of learning wasn't your style. Now, though, you can learn *your* way. Personally, I delved into the career that had dropped into my lap and took courses on coaching, podcast editing, and small-business development. I attended Bible studies and networking groups. I read about a variety of topics, including personal healing, spiritual growth, and productivity. With each course I took, each book I read, and each skill I explored or developed, I felt stronger and more capable. It didn't happen overnight; remember, this is a long game. But the process is gratifying and the results are oh-so-worth it.

Practicalities

Getting all the "necessaries" settled can be overwhelming, to put it mildly. Somehow, I muddled through setting up bank accounts, updating my will, obtaining insurance, filing taxes, and so on—*and you will too*. Once the dust settles, you may even find it empowering. But it's hard to focus on to-do lists, as important as they are, when your emotions are a hot mess. To assist with that, I recommend a book called *Your Post-Divorce Compass* by Michael R. Dunham, a smart and supportive family lawyer I met in a business networking group. Mike outlines simple but necessary steps, one per day, to help you get your new life in order. His book is worth the price in peace of mind alone. (You can find more informationon in the Recommended Resources section at the end of this book.)

Travel

It's easy to have a scarcity mindset when you're facing a divorce or are recently divorced. By all means, carefully budget and be intentional about your spending. But don't forget the healing that comes with getting out into the world and immersing yourself in the beauty and variety of God's creation. If there's any way you can swing it, "gettin' outta Dodge" for a while will contribute to your self-care during this time.

Visit old friends. Take a day trip to a place you've always wanted to see. Hit the road and stop at all the visitors centers and/or tourist areas (the brown highway signs) you come across. Meet new people. These activities will help you remember that life isn't *all* about what's happening to you right now. If you can manage it in the future, pull out your calendar and schedule a trip once or twice a year. It will not only give you something fun to anticipate, but you'll also start building a stock of new, happier memories.

Two stories bookend this truth in my life.

A few months before my divorce was finalized, a woman I'd met online and become friends with was on a road trip, stopping for a few days at a beach about a three-hour drive from my home. We'd hit it off from the time we met and had grown close over the years. We were both authors and homeschool veterans, had co-hosted a podcast together, and were in similar life stages. The weekend she was at the beach, my kids from out of town were visiting. We were enjoying our time together, but as we were sitting on the couch, I got a text from my friend inviting me to come visit her. My crazy middle son saw it, grabbed my phone, and responded. (Don't worry; I talk about boundaries in Chapter 5.) Pretending to be me, he wrote, "Yes, text me your address—I'll be on my way!" *What!!* I started to chastise him and argue, but almost in one voice, my kids encouraged me to go. They'd see me again, they reasoned, but when would I get another chance to meet my friend in *my* neck of the woods? So off I went.

And I will never forget the gratitude, independence, optimism, and empowerment I felt on the road. It was truly a gift, one that bolstered my heart during the dark days that were still to come.

Then, about six months after my divorce, my elder daughter and son-in-law invited me to accompany them on a trip to the Poconos. They were exploring opportunities to purchase rental real estate, and I think they both thought a change of scenery would be helpful to me.

They were right.

Sitting outside in the early fall, watching colorful leaves float down from the trees, I had an "aha moment." It gave me a new perspective on the season of life I'd found myself in. It helped me to reframe my disappointment and pain, and to understand that God was indeed laying a foundation for my future.

A snippet from a short story I wrote about the experience may clarify that concept:

> Does autumn ever look at the leaves on the ground and wonder, "What did I do wrong?"
>
> Does Mother Nature look around at the barren trees in the winter with disappointment and ask, "Hey, what happened here?"
>
> I sat and pondered these questions over a glass of wine as I thoughtfully reviewed the past year. (Okay, maybe it was the second glass that got me asking those questions, but still.) …
>
> Why do we look at the inevitable changes in our lives and immediately assume that something went wrong when there is the slightest bit of pain, discomfort, or disorder? That we

messed up somewhere? That we "missed the memo" or somehow took a wrong turn?

A few days later, seated amid the falling leaves in my backyard, I saw a Facebook post from a friend of mine. The gorgeous photos of Michigan trees at their peak of color, along with her comment, seemed to sum up my conclusions:

"Take it as you wish, but basically, it all boils down to the fact that God is good in every season. Maybe dreams don't really die, maybe they fade, fall, and feed into the bigger dreams yet to be sown."

What a beautiful bookend to my fall thoughts! ... a confirmation that even the worst of the preceding years could be framed more positively.

What a clear visual image to recall when feeling tempted to entertain a pity party or thinking the dreams of the past were dead and the events of the past brought only despair.[4]

Had I stayed home with the covers pulled over my head, stewing in my personal pity party, I would never have received such a beautiful visual image to encourage my future growth.

If taking care of yourself is a new thing, let me gently remind you that everyone's journey is different, so don't compare yourself to anyone else. If you have a competitive personality streak and feel compelled to do so, journal about your "personal bests" or accomplishments along the way. When you look back over your words someday, you'll be proud of how far you've come. (And if you need help getting started with self-care, head over to Chapter 14 for some quick wins.)

YOUR TURN

Start creating a detailed self-care plan. If that's too overwhelming, what is *one* thing you will do this week to take care of yourself?

3.
R: Rebuild Trust

"The Lord is my strength and my shield; my heart trusts in Him and He helps me." ~ Psalm 28:7

"Fool me once, shame on you. Fool me twice, shame on me." ~ Anthony Weldon

Rebuilding trust—whether in others or your own instincts, feelings and abilities—is one of the most difficult things to do after a marriage fails. Whether you've been fooled once or a thousand times—by infidelity, deceit, gaslighting, or abuse—you feel uniquely hurt and raw and exposed.

Few of us go into marriage planning to keep secrets, expecting to be hurt, or anticipating disappointment. It takes a deep commitment and vulnerability to risk being our true selves with another person when we're anticipating a lifelong relationship. So when that trust is broken, it cuts to the core.

Unfortunately, there is no quick fix for this problem. Relational trust is neither easily nor quickly rebuilt, and I won't mislead you by giving you six simple steps or twelve guaranteed strategies to help you be a tower of strength and a trusting human being in thirty days or less. I can, however, share some principles to keep in mind as you navigate this season.

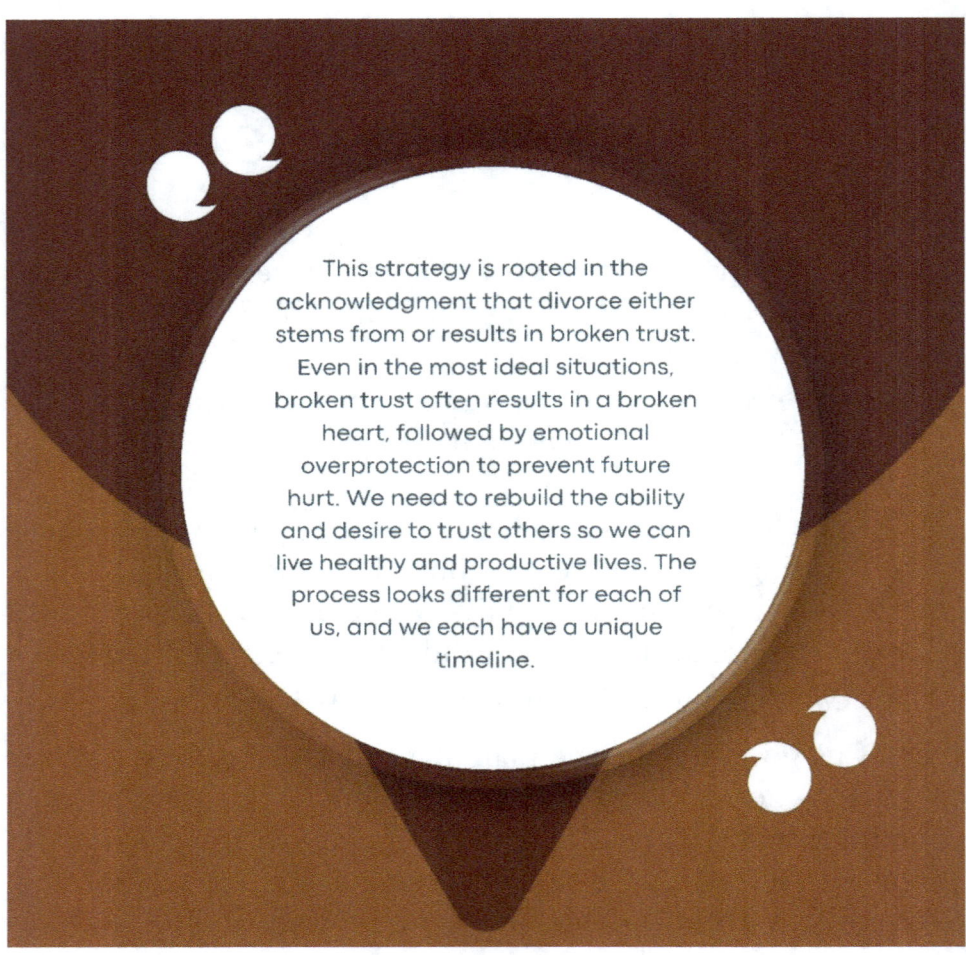

This strategy is rooted in the acknowledgment that divorce either stems from or results in broken trust. Even in the most ideal situations, broken trust often results in a broken heart, followed by emotional overprotection to prevent future hurt. We need to rebuild the ability and desire to trust others so we can live healthy and productive lives. The process looks different for each of us, and we each have a unique timeline.

Trust is important because it is the glue that holds relationships together. An article in *Psychology Today* offers a fantastic summary of the benefits of trust and explains how critical it is in our personal and business relationships, as well as in society in general. The bottom line is this: "People who trust each other can work together more effectively at home, at work, or elsewhere. They are also more willing to share intimate information, which can reduce the risk of anxiety and depression and build a stronger sense of self."[5]

Trauma can damage trust, however, and divorce is often a cause of trauma, no matter how "friendly" or mutually agreed upon the divorce is. So how does one begin to heal from the broken trust that results from divorce?

First and foremost, don't rush this phase. You'll read this caveat multiple times in this book because it's that important. Some people will risk vulnerability sooner because they are naturally trusting. They may have a strong need to have a close relationship and quickly fill the void left by their divorce, which doesn't necessarily fix the problems that led to the initial divorce.

The key is to take care of yourself in a healthy way (see Chapter 2), allow yourself time to grieve, and then move ahead at your own pace. It's neither a race nor a competition, so to borrow a directive from the Bible, "look neither to the left nor to the right" as you proceed.[6] God has a plan for you, and keeping focused on your own life will help you stay steady as you move forward.

Remember we're all human. Being in any relationship guarantees you'll be hurt and disappointed at some point. That applies whether it's a romantic relationship or with friends, colleagues, or adult children. But don't forget this goes both ways—you're bound to hurt and disappoint others at one point or another too. So practice empathy. Offer people the benefit of the doubt. Give the grace to others that you know you'll probably need from them someday. Realize that we're all doing the best we can, and sometimes others may not meet our needs. But at the end of the day, the world doesn't exist to meet our needs anyway.

Start small. Once you do feel ready to look for another relationship, start with finding a friend. Early in my divorce, I did not want to meet anyone. Serious or not, male or female, friend or lover—I was *so* "not looking." I remember visiting churches after I moved, going in and out without so much as a "good morning" to anyone. I avoided eye contact like the plague. I finally forced myself to go swing dancing with my elder daughter because I like music, and I could be social without really getting to know anyone. (You do what you can do, right? While I wasn't ready for a relationship, I realized I *did* need to have some fun.)

Navigate new relationships carefully. Once you are ready for dating, let me emphasize two realities you may have already discovered. First, it's a different dating world out there! Because of our age and perhaps the length of our marriages, we may not have been on a date with someone other than a spouse since we were in college or just starting out in the workforce. Most likely it was during the 1960s, 70s, 80s, or even 90s—long before dating apps, in other words. Boy, talk about perspective! Also, adult friendships, let alone serious relationships, can be hard. Because of social media and our lack of privacy, it's so much easier to get scammed or be taken advantage of. When you do meet someone, make sure you manage your expectations and communicate them well. Do whatever you need to maintain your (perhaps) newfound sense of self, and establish safe and healthy boundaries.

Seek help. No matter what side of the "vs." you're on in the divorce papers, the whole process of dissolving a life together, separating finances, parsing out property, and dealing with hurt children (of any age) and confused friends is a lot to manage. A good counselor can help you heal well, rebuild trust, and craft a life better than you could ever imagine. Along the way, you might also be able to

organize your thoughts,

gain perspective,

understand yourself better,

talk in a judgment-free zone, and

be challenged to grow in a safe space.[7]

As a Christian, my saving grace was prayer. I understood divorce is a process, but receiving the final decree that made me newly single again left me reeling. I realized that no matter how close I would ever again be with someone, the only One who would never disappoint me, who would always have my back, and who I could always trust, was God. I sought and went through Bible studies that focused on the names of God, the promises of God, and the characteristics of God. At a time when it would have been easy to turn my back on Him, I dug deep and determined that He alone could be trusted to provide whatever I needed to get through this and come out better on the other side.

He didn't disappoint me either.

Here is a partial list of the biblical promises I found helpful as I started this exercise:

"Be strong and of good courage, do not fear nor be afraid of them; for the LORD your God, He is the One who goes with you. He will not leave you nor forsake you." ~ Deuteronomy 31:6

"I have blotted out, like a thick cloud, your transgressions, and like a cloud, your sins. Return to Me, for I have redeemed you." ~ Isaiah 44:22

"I will instruct you and teach you in the way you should go; I will guide you with My eye." ~ Psalm 32:8

"For He satisfies the longing soul, and fills the hungry soul with goodness." ~ Psalm 107:9

"For God has not given us a spirit of fear, but of power and of love and of a sound mind." ~ 2 Timothy 1:7

"When I said. 'My foot is slipping,' your unfailing love, Lord, supported me." ~ Psalm 94:18

YOUR TURN
What is the first step you'll take as you begin to trust again?

4.
E: Expect the Best

"We tend to get what we expect."
~ Norman Vincent Peale

"My happiness grows in direct proportion to my acceptance, and in inverse proportion to my expectations."
~ Michael J. Fox

Have you ever heard of a superbloom? It happens in the desert every five to ten years or so. After years of arid weather, the conditions are such that long-dormant seeds spring to life. The result is a breathtaking expanse of color and variety so dense and wide-ranging that it often can be seen from space.[8]

Superblooms result from a perfect storm of requirements. Most notable (and applicable here) are the presence of dormant seeds underground and an abundance of consistent rain.

I was introduced to this phenomenon a few months after my divorce became final. I had already started my business, but I remained doubtful I could ever *really* support myself. Each day seemed to bring more than its fair share of rain. Insecurity and depression were doing their best to encourage the seeds of self-pity, self-doubt, and fear to grow.

Thankfully, my adult kids rallied around me, planting seeds to counteract the weeds lying in wait. A new perfect storm was brewing as I implemented the principles and strategies in this book. Through prayer, persistence, counsel, and grace, these new seeds developed roots and began to grow. I started to feel a glimmer of hope as I saw the potential for a beautiful future. Imagine: *a superbloom in my own life!*

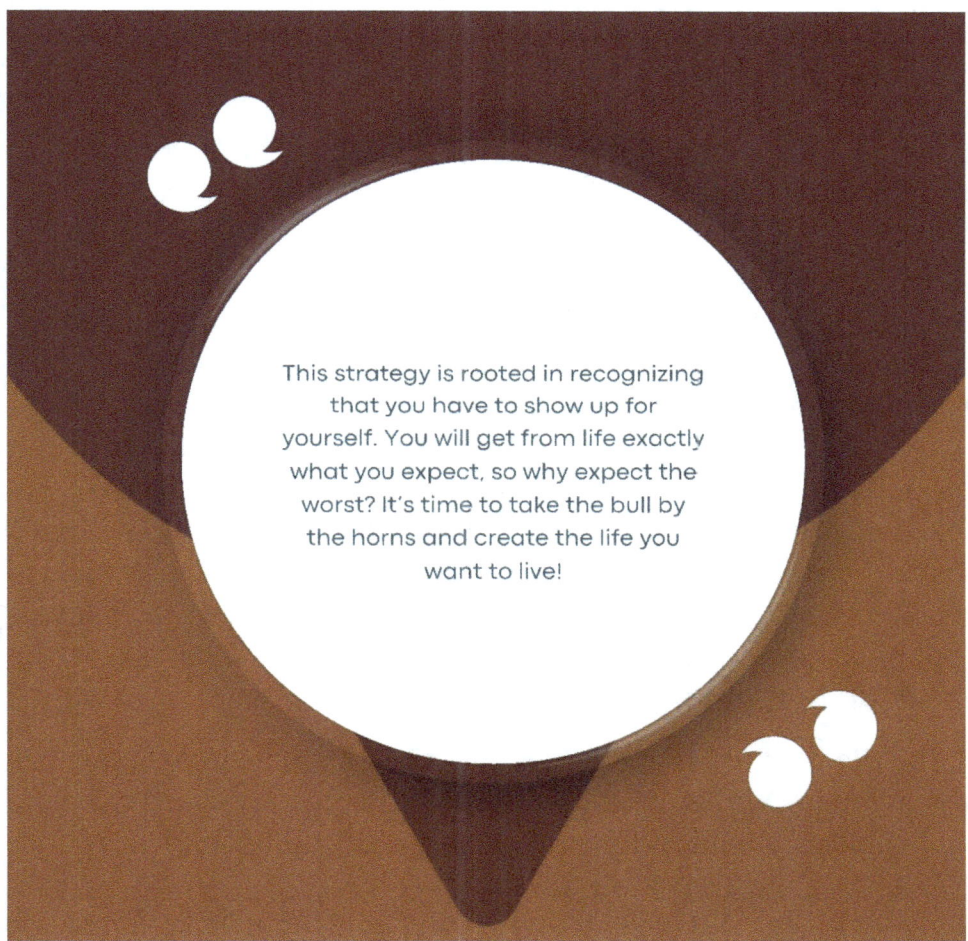

This strategy is rooted in recognizing that you have to show up for yourself. You will get from life exactly what you expect, so why expect the worst? It's time to take the bull by the horns and create the life you want to live!

I knew I had to take action. I needed to show up for myself because, married or not, that was never anyone else's job, anyway. I began to develop what one of my daughters called "relentless optimism."

I no longer had the luxury of seeing the glass half empty. I couldn't waste my time playing the "what-if" game with an attitude of negativity. Being realistic is fine, but I realized that when I viewed things through a pessimistic lens, negativity was all I would ever see.

I was in crisis, and *I* was responsible for getting myself out of it. Clearly, I needed to adjust my approach to life and begin to manage my expectations.

I love the perspective that Michael J. Fox's quote at the beginning of this chapter brings to the concept of expectations. While it's okay to expect the best of people or situations, it's just as important that we are not tied to the *outcome*. In other words, we must accept things as they are and not be rigid about the result or end game. When we hold our plans, hopes, and dreams with open hands, we're more likely to appreciate what we already have, be centered in the "now," and be amused by unexpected outcomes. We are better able to maintain a delicate balance of optimism and reality and become better able to focus on and be grateful for the present.

"The Parable of the Farmer and the Horse" (also known as "Maybe So, Maybe Not") is a great example of how maintaining a balanced mindset toward events enables us to learn from whatever experiences we have.[9]

The story tells of a farmer whose horse escapes, prompting his neighbors to lament his misfortune. The farmer responds calmly, "Perhaps, perhaps not." The following day, the horse returns, along with several other wild horses. The neighbors celebrate his good luck, but the farmer again says, "Perhaps, perhaps not." Later, while attempting to tame one of the wild horses, the farmer's son falls and breaks his leg. The neighbors again express their sympathy for this setback, and the farmer repeats, "Perhaps, perhaps not." Not long after, the army arrives in the village to draft young men for war but spares the farmer's son because of his injury. The neighbors remark on the fortunate turn of events, and the farmer replies with the usual, "Perhaps, perhaps not."

This tale illustrates the ever-changing nature of circumstances, emphasizing that events we perceive as either positive or negative may shift over time. Applying this perspective in our own lives can help us embrace the lessons from our experiences without rigidly categorizing them as "good" or "bad," allowing us to grow and evolve.

Specifically, we can reframe our life perspective post-divorce. I did it, and I know you can do it too.

YOUR TURN

What action or actions will you take to begin to expect the best from yourself? Of others? Of life?

5.
N: Know Your Boundaries

"Boundaries are like fences: they keep out what you don't want and protect what you value." ~ Henry Cloud

"Boundaries define our outer limits and protect our inner peace." ~ Brené Brown

Many years ago, we built what we imagined was our dream home. The main floor had a kitchen and dining room that opened to the living room, which featured a fireplace, a two-story high ceiling, and windows all around. The upstairs had a loft area and three bedrooms that opened to a hallway overlooking the living room. Whenever I cooked or baked, the house would fill with sweet or savory aromas. The kids loved playing in the loft, and I enjoyed hearing happy giggles whenever they were up to their shenanigans. However, whenever any of us wanted to have a private conversation, we were compelled to go outside on the porch (not exactly ideal during summers in southwest Georgia), talk in the master bedroom (not always appropriate), or head downstairs to the partially finished basement.

We soon realized the error of our ways. Turns out, an open floor plan with few boundaries wasn't our dream home after all. Although we enjoyed our years there, it was a welcome relief to later move into a smaller house with a more traditional floor plan.

Boundaries are like that.

They provide spaces in which we can fully enjoy activities and time with loved ones. They define areas and times in our lives which—although it seems counter-intuitive—allow us to live a freer life. When we are clear with our boundaries, we love and serve others without resentment or rancor. When we communicate our boundaries well, both parties benefit from mutual understanding, and healthy relationships can flourish.

As I mentioned in an earlier chapter, boundaries are not demanding specific behaviors from others or defining how you want them to behave. For example, "Stop talking like that to me!" or "Don't do that anymore" doesn't qualify as boundary setting. Rather, boundaries are sharing what you will do in response to a specific behavior. For instance, "If you say that to me again, I'll stop talking to you," or "If you do (such and such) to me, I will not hang out with you." See the difference?

I wish I understood this concept years ago.

I grew up and entered my marriage believing I was *always* expected to consider others' needs above my own. That any need I might feel for private time or personal space was selfish and sinful. That any bitterness or resentment I felt was best prayed over, asking God to remove those feelings from my life. I got so wrapped up in trying to be a good mother and wife that I forgot about myself.

I don't recommend living that way.

As a Christian, I spent a lot of time praying about the idea of boundaries. I began to see that even Jesus had them (not that I'm comparing myself to Him). Even He went alone into the desert to pray. For various reasons, He sometimes withheld time and attention from his family and disciples—the people closest to him on this earth. When His dear friend Lazarus died, Jesus made Lazarus's sisters wait two days before He went to visit and comfort them. He waited because He could see the bigger picture, and He wanted to showcase God's extravagant love for His friends.

On numerous occasions, when tempted by men or Satan, Jesus withdrew when He realized their only intent was to trap Him. He protected His prayer time and treasured longer moments to be alone with the Father. Setting boundaries helped Him guard His values and fulfill His mission.[10]

If my Savior needed time apart, surely that's good enough for me.

It's perfectly healthy, normal, *and necessary* to have and honor margin in your life through establishing healthy boundaries.

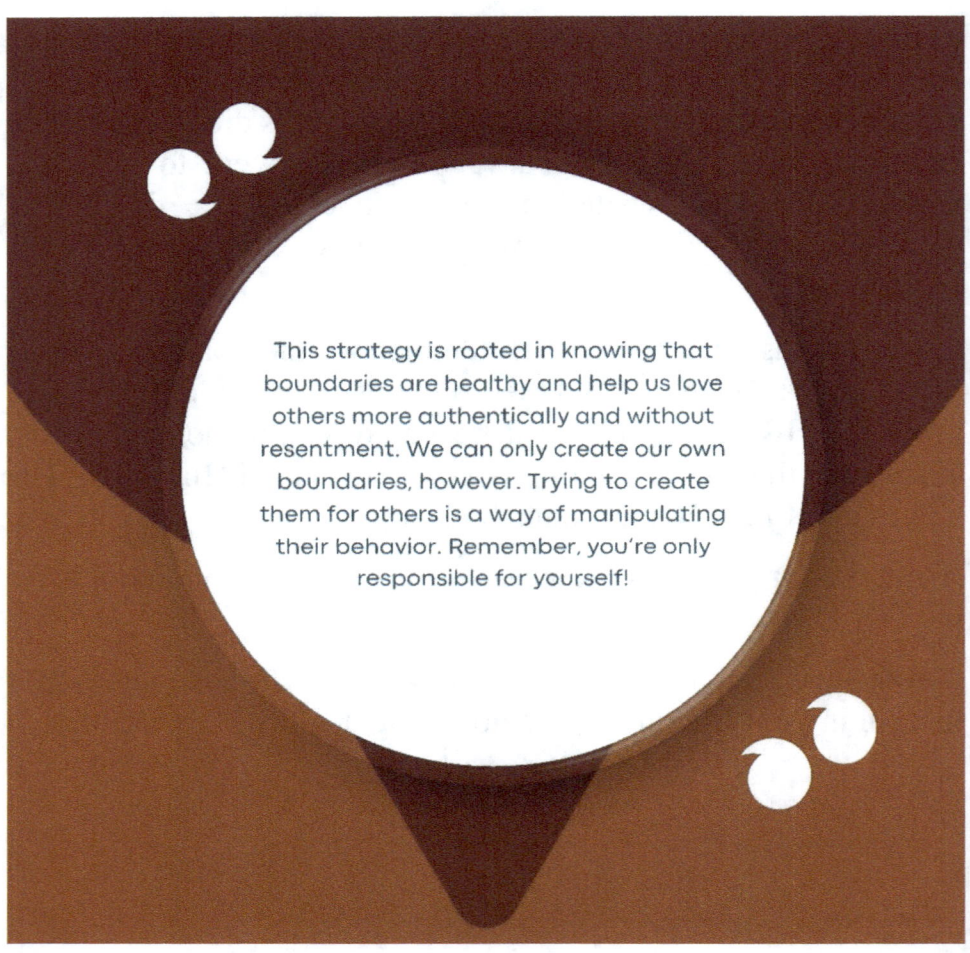

This strategy is rooted in knowing that boundaries are healthy and help us love others more authentically and without resentment. We can only create our own boundaries, however. Trying to create them for others is a way of manipulating their behavior. Remember, you're only responsible for yourself!

Shortly before my divorce was finalized, I moved from South Carolina to Atlanta to be closer to my adult kids and their growing families. I had many happy memories of my grandparents' involvement in my life as I was growing up. Years later, my mother-in-law enjoyed many years of living near us and watching our kids grow up. I wanted to be a bigger part of my children's and grandchildren's lives too. I blissfully imagined babysitting often, popping in to say hi, or sharing meals or activities regularly. But I also had to support myself. And relearn how to drive in traffic. And build a brand new life that included making friends, finding a church, learning home repair skills, and so on.

I needed to establish boundaries with my time and availability. I had to learn how to say no rather than twist myself into a pretzel to serve my children and their families. I needed to be able to disappoint them from time to time when our schedules didn't allow for getting together. I began to understand that even though I wanted to be more involved with their lives, that didn't mean I couldn't have a life, time, things to do, and events to attend without them.

Maybe you're saying, "Well, duh!" But it was a revelation to me after years of codependency.

So, my friend, now it's time to look at your life. Where do you need to establish boundaries? Maybe that's too big of a question to start with. Maybe, as we discussed in Chapter 2, you need to get to know yourself better. Here are a few questions to help you get started:

- What do you enjoy doing? Boundary: Make time to engage in those activities and make it non-negotiable.

- Do you work for yourself from home? Boundary: Set work hours, stick to them (which you'd have to do if you were employed at an office anyway), and communicate them to the people in your life.

- What's a skill or hobby you've always wanted to learn or try? Boundary: Find training for it, sign up, and see it through. Again, make the necessary time for training and practice non-negotiable.

- Establish emotional boundaries too. Is there a topic you are working through in counseling or you're still healing from? Summon the confidence to inform others that it's off limits for discussion with you right now.

Learning, setting, and sticking to boundaries is a form of self-care. Boundaries allow you to serve and love people from a full cup, rather than an empty one. It may be hard to learn, but if you're on this journey of healing and recovery, think of it as a gift.

You're getting to create a life of freedom filled with choices. Allow boundaries to help you.

YOUR TURN

What boundaries do you need to create or maintain so that you can love others authentically and have a healthy life?

6.
G: BE GENTLE WITH YOURSELF

"Talk to yourself the way you would to someone you love."
~ Brené Brown

"The love and attention you always thought you wanted from someone else is the love and attention you first need to give to yourself."
~ Bryant McGill

Even before the ink dried on the final paperwork, I felt the urgency to "get my act together." At the ripe old age of 60, I was starting from scratch. I looked around and saw married family members, friends, and colleagues—all around my same age—preparing for retirement, enjoying grandkids, and planning vacations or traveling together. Some were downsizing with the eager anticipation of a simpler life.

I, on the other hand, had very little saved for retirement, and the weight of feeling ill-prepared was heavy on my shoulders. While I *was* looking forward to spending time with my grandchildren, my downsizing was necessary (and a tad stressful) because of my financial and employment situation (see Chapter 10). I faced a never-ending to-do list, and not a day went by that I didn't feel overwhelmed, mentally and emotionally exhausted, and super stressed about the looming future.

It was a complete recipe for burnout.

Somehow, I had to drum up the wherewithal to manage all the details of my new life: finding a place to live, starting a business, establishing bank and credit card accounts in my name, and so on. I continued to push through—mostly out of fear and panic—and sheer adrenaline kept me going through each day.

Things eventually started to settle down, however. After a few months, my revamped affairs seemed to be in order.

Life slowed down and I became quiet enough to hear my own voice talking to me. But it wasn't very nice.

Ha! You think you can keep this up?

You haven't had to support yourself since just after college—what makes you think you can do it now?

You don't have any retirement savings. What happens if you get a major illness or can't work anymore?

Your ex already has a new relationship—you'll probably end up old and lonely.

After years of being excessively hard on myself, after years of distracting myself when I was being too self-critical, I had finally hit the wall.

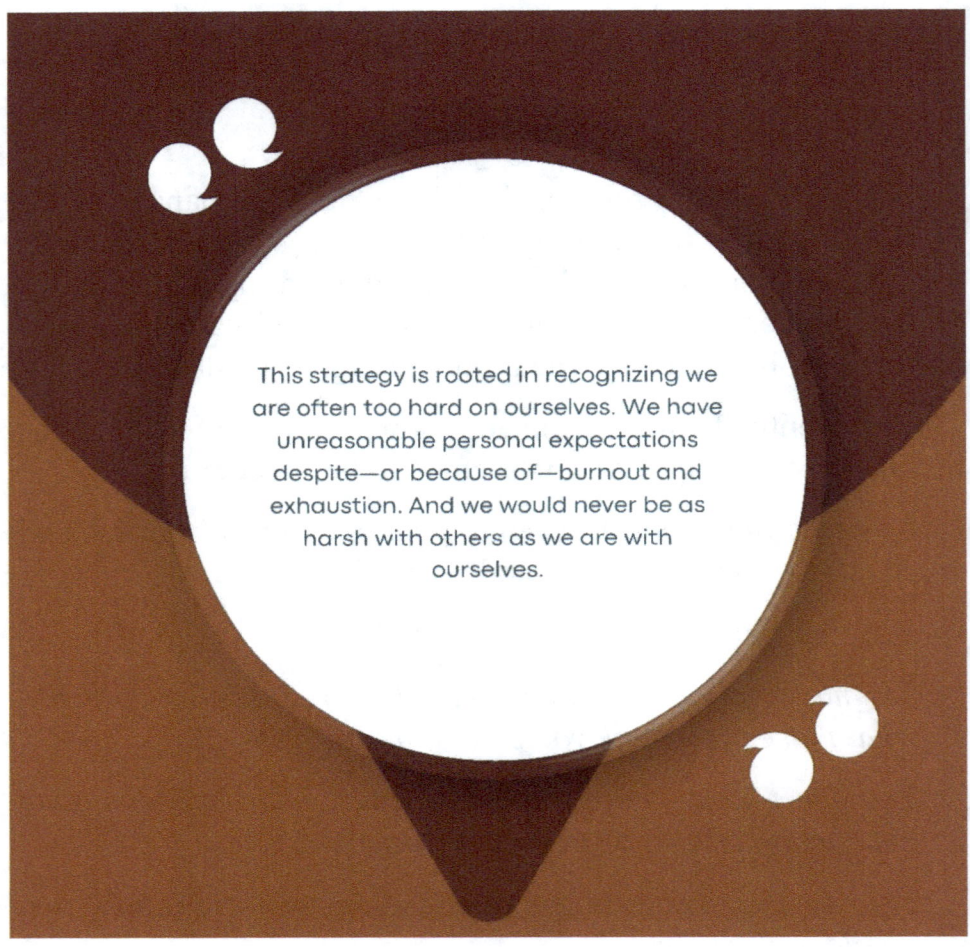

This strategy is rooted in recognizing we are often too hard on ourselves. We have unreasonable personal expectations despite—or because of—burnout and exhaustion. And we would never be as harsh with others as we are with ourselves.

We are most susceptible to being hard on ourselves when we are tired, disappointed, or burned out. That's because when we're at our worst, our emotions take over and we equate what we feel with reality. Whatever we're feeling is usually negative, which makes us approach reality from that perspective. This is understandable, but what makes it even worse is that we may have developed a habit of negative self-talk over the years and aren't even aware of it. People who tend to be the most in danger of this are those with Type A personalities, eldest children, Enneagram Type 1s, and individuals who were raised by supercritical parents or spent years being gaslit in relationships.

But, yes, this also applies to almost anyone with a beating heart. And it didn't take me long to realize constantly beating myself up was no way to live.

Looking back, I'm so grateful God led me to just the right resources. I'm not surprised, though. The way I see it, this is yet another example of those divinely directed "coincidences" we talked about in the Introduction. And you remember how I feel about *them*, right?

The right resources are only part of the solution, however. Even with those in place, the very necessary strategy of being gentle with ourselves takes a boatload of work. I'll share a bit of my journey so you can see what it might entail for you.

- I began counseling again. (We had been through years of marriage counseling, but this was just for me.). This helped me discover the root of my bad habit of being so hard on myself, but I soon realized it wasn't enough simply to know where this came from if I was going to get in front of it.

- So I moved on to mindset coaching. I found a terrific life coach who is a Christian. She helped me explore my strengths and reframe my internal conversations. I began to develop a more balanced, healthy, and reasonable approach to myself, where I was coming from, and what I was dealing with.

- I dug into my faith and relationship with God, which reignited my prayer life and connection to something and Someone bigger than myself.

- I found an intellectually stimulating church where I could serve others and thus get my focus off *my* problems.

- I crafted a vision and a set of business-related values so I could have a more synergistic life. (Solopreneurs and small-business owners know exactly what I'm talking about here.)

The result—which is still and will always be a work in progress—was a life that feels more balanced than it ever did. I slowed down and realized I wasn't responsible for *everything*, even though I was now single (see Chapter 1). I began to take better care of myself (see Chapter 2). I stopped comparing myself to others (see Chapter 3). I started to expect more out of life (see Chapter 4). And I began to set and navigate personal boundaries (see Chapter 5).

Being gentle with yourself doesn't mean you allow yourself to stay in bed all day. It doesn't mean you binge Netflix or stick your hand in a family size bag of chips or cookies and have at it. You can still challenge yourself. You can still encourage yourself to stretch beyond what you think you can do and attempt bigger things you once only imagined.

Being gentle with yourself means you keep the end in mind: becoming a whole and healthy person. It means you parent the hurt child that may emerge in your heart because of this experience. It means you learn—or relearn—all the skills you may have taught your own children with the intention of helping them grow into happy, functioning adults with thriving relationships.

Use these strategies and concepts to help *yourself* move forward. But remember: You're going through a personal battle, so make sure you use them with kid gloves.

YOUR TURN
What's one thing you need to back off of to be more gentle with yourself?

7.
T: BE THANKFUL

"Gratitude turns whatever we have into enough."
~ Unknown

"Gratitude is not only the greatest of virtues but the parent of all others."
~ Cicero

"The more grateful I am, the more beauty I see."
~ Mary Davis

Of all the strategies and mindset adjustments in this book, this one was the most challenging for me. It's not something that comes naturally to most of us, and certainly not at a time when we're trying to heal from a traumatic life experience. That said, when we're practicing gratitude, it retrains our mind and—thanks to neuroplasticity—literally rewires our brains to look for things for which we can be grateful. Fortunately, I had heard someone mention this a long time ago, so when I found a sign at Hobby Lobby that said "Gratitude Turns Whatever We Have Into Enough," I snagged it. (This, despite finding myself smack dab in the middle of a bout of self-pity and feeling hypocritical and inauthentic for making the purchase.)

I hung it in the hall opposite the door to my office. Some days, when I was feeling less grateful, I wouldn't even glance at it. But more and more, I found myself using it as a prompt to make myself think of "just one thing" to give thanks for. I took the easy route at first. For example, every day for five days, I'd pick *one* of my five children to be thankful for (no, I'm not kidding). It became easier over time, though, and as I continued to challenge myself, I began identifying *two* blessings each day. Once I got up to three, I started a notepad on my phone and would record them each morning before my feet hit the floor. At the time of this writing, I've done this for ten straight months. And I've been surprised to discover that I rarely repeat myself. Turns out, the more I make a habit of looking for things to be grateful for, the easier it becomes to keep finding more. Coincidence? I think not.

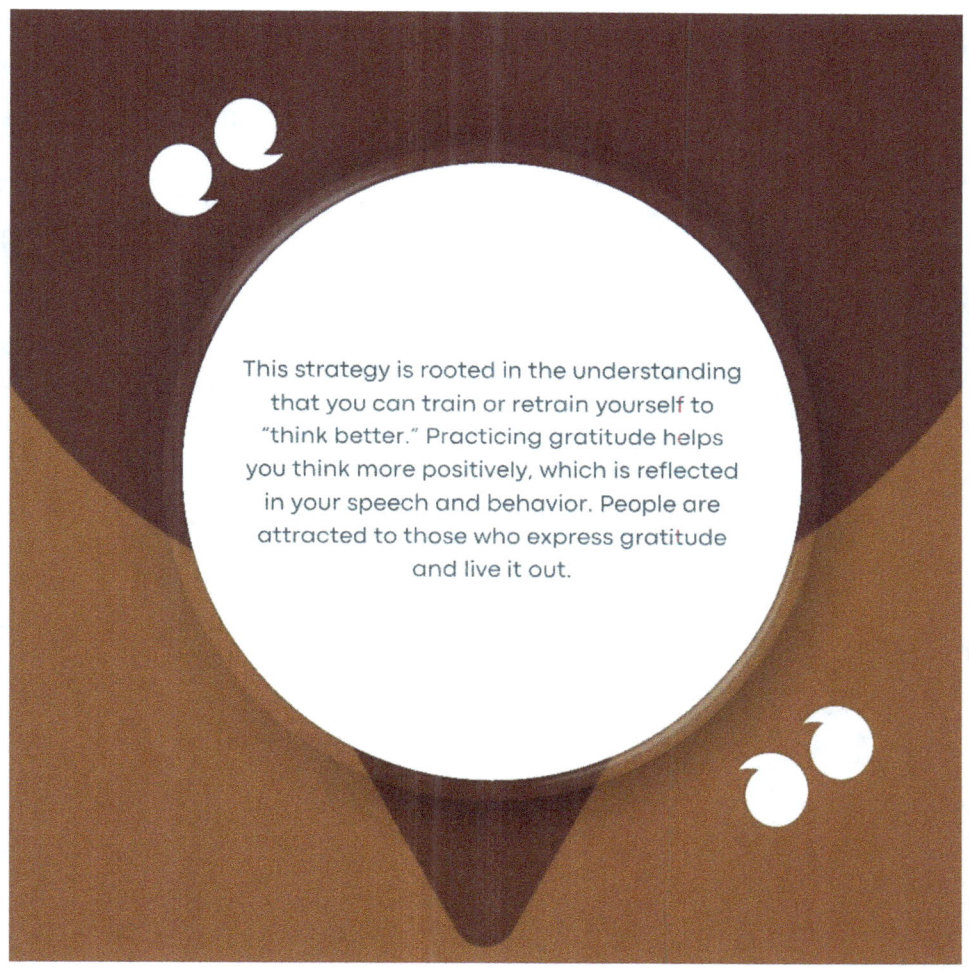

This strategy is rooted in the understanding that you can train or retrain yourself to "think better." Practicing gratitude helps you think more positively, which is reflected in your speech and behavior. People are attracted to those who express gratitude and live it out.

I should add that there have been days when finding something to be thankful for was a chore. On one of my more difficult days, I wrote, "1.—sleeping in on a weekday, 2.—safety on the highway last night, 3.—grapefruit juice." Not exactly inspiring, I know. But there have been other days when I'd start writing in the morning or keep my notepad open all day and get up to twelve or fifteen items.

Particularly on days when I had a session with my life coach or counselor, I found it easier to be aware of all the people, things, and events for which I'm grateful. (One more benefit of seeking professional help, I suppose.)

Working on my mindset is always a work in progress, and I now understand that being positive and optimistic takes intentional practice. Practice makes perfect, friend—or at least it gets easier!

YOUR TURN
Grab a clean, small notebook and begin to write *one* thing you're grateful for each day. Build up to two or three. Wash, rinse, and repeat!

8.
H: Have a Sense of Humor

"If you could choose one characteristic that would get you through life, choose a sense of humor."
~ Jennifer Jones

"A cheerful heart is good medicine, but a broken spirit saps a person's strength."
~ Proverbs 17:22 (NLT)

The power of laughter has long been recognized in both medicine and faith.[12] As for me? Well, as the song from the musical *Mary Poppins* puts it, I *love* to laugh!

My favorite times these days are when I get together with my adult kiddos. My three youngest have this spark of humor among them that fans into a flame if they're in the same room for more than a minute. When we're all together, they turn it up even higher.

No topic is out of bounds, and the laughs just keep coming. I often find myself struggling to catch my breath, or with tears streaming down my face, or (considering the season of life I'm in) finding it necessary to, um, visit the little girls' room!

I always feel better when my children are around.

In the evenings, I enjoy watching the clean comedians on Dry Bar Comedy; some of them are just amazing. And don't even get me started on all the funny movies, sitcoms from the 1980s and 90s, books, podcasts, and internet memes—there's a treasure trove of humor out there, just waiting to help you heal.

Now I'm *not* suggesting that watching a funny movie or laughing with friends is going to make everything alright. But I *am* saying that a good belly laugh every now and then takes your mind off the pain of the day and allows you to refocus, reframe, and readjust your perspective on life.

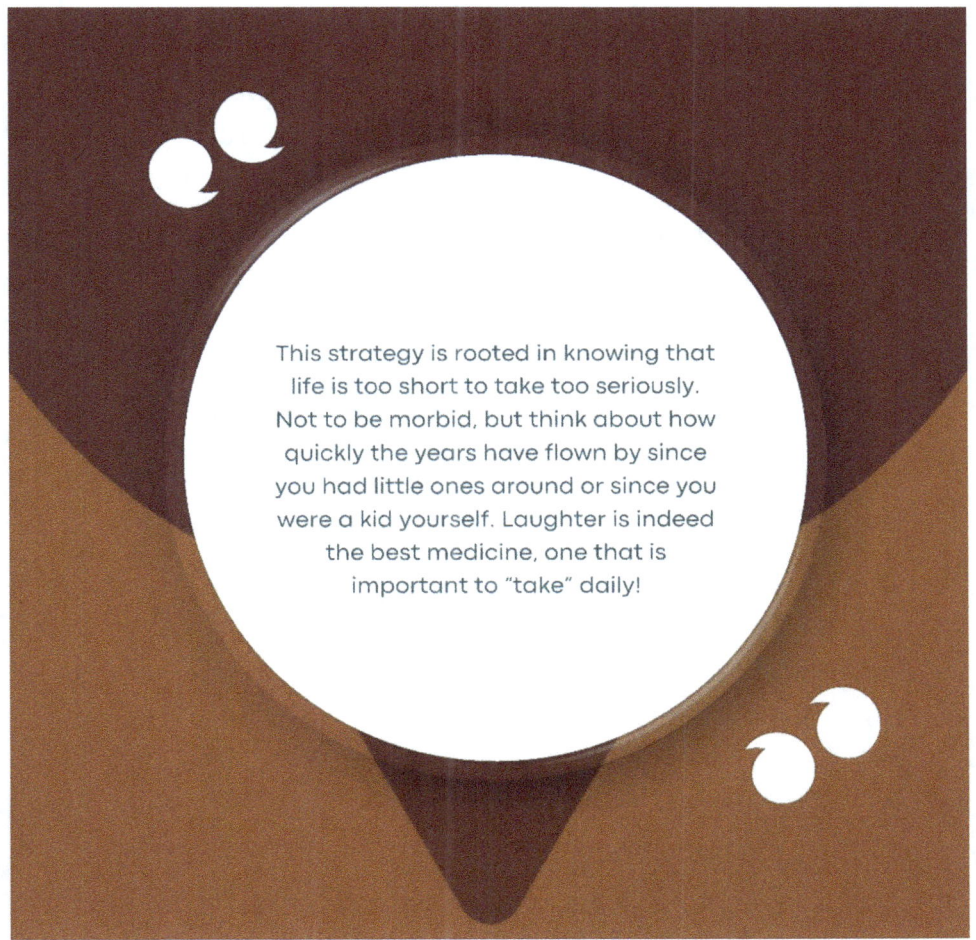

This strategy is rooted in knowing that life is too short to take too seriously. Not to be morbid, but think about how quickly the years have flown by since you had little ones around or since you were a kid yourself. Laughter is indeed the best medicine, one that is important to "take" daily!

A close friend of mine took this strategy to the extreme and enrolled in a course on stand-up comedy. To be fair, she *is* a riot, with a natural sense of humor. I always feel better after being around her for a while. She had a great time taking the class; she met some interesting people and it stretched her comfort zone. She also learned that being funny and making it your job isn't quite the same thing. But hey, nothing ventured, nothing gained, right? At the very least, it was a terrific experience, she has some hilarious stories, and it makes for a great conversation starter.

Take some time right now to think about what makes you laugh. If that's too big of a stretch, think about some things that bring a smile to your face. Write them down so you can refer to your list from time to time.

When life gets too heavy to carry, put that load down and grab some laughs instead.

YOUR TURN

What makes you laugh? If you don't know, try something new every day until you find what it is that tickles your funny bone. Then incorporate that one thing into your day every day!

_____
_____
_____
_____
_____
_____
_____
_____
_____
_____
_____
_____
_____
_____
_____
_____
_____
_____

9.
S: Show Forgiveness

"Unforgiveness is like taking poison and waiting for the other person to die."
~ Marianne Wilkerson

"When you forgive, you in no way change the past. But you sure do change the future."
~ Bernard Meltzer

Note: Please note that this is an "advanced" stop on the path to divorce recovery. You might not be here yet, and I don't want to hurt you further or set you back. Read this chapter when you have had or are in the process of personal counseling and are on the road to healing.

Ah, forgiveness—so easy to talk about, so easy to suggest, so easy to recommend, and so hard to do!

Although the act of forgiveness can make you feel as if you're taking years off your age (which it may or may not do) or pounds off your frame (which it most likely does *not* do), it *does* take that proverbial chip off your shoulder, which is decidedly wonderful. But the flip side of the coin is news you may not want to hear: Forgiveness is an ongoing process.

Every so often, despite thinking I've "arrived" and totally forgiven my ex, something triggers me, and—there I go again—feelings of anger, sadness, disappointment, hurt, or _____ (fill in the blank here with your nasty feeling du jour) pop up, and I realize I have to do it all over again.

Forgive, that is.

But let me encourage you that it's worth it. (Okay, to be transparent, let me encourage *myself* that it's worth it.)

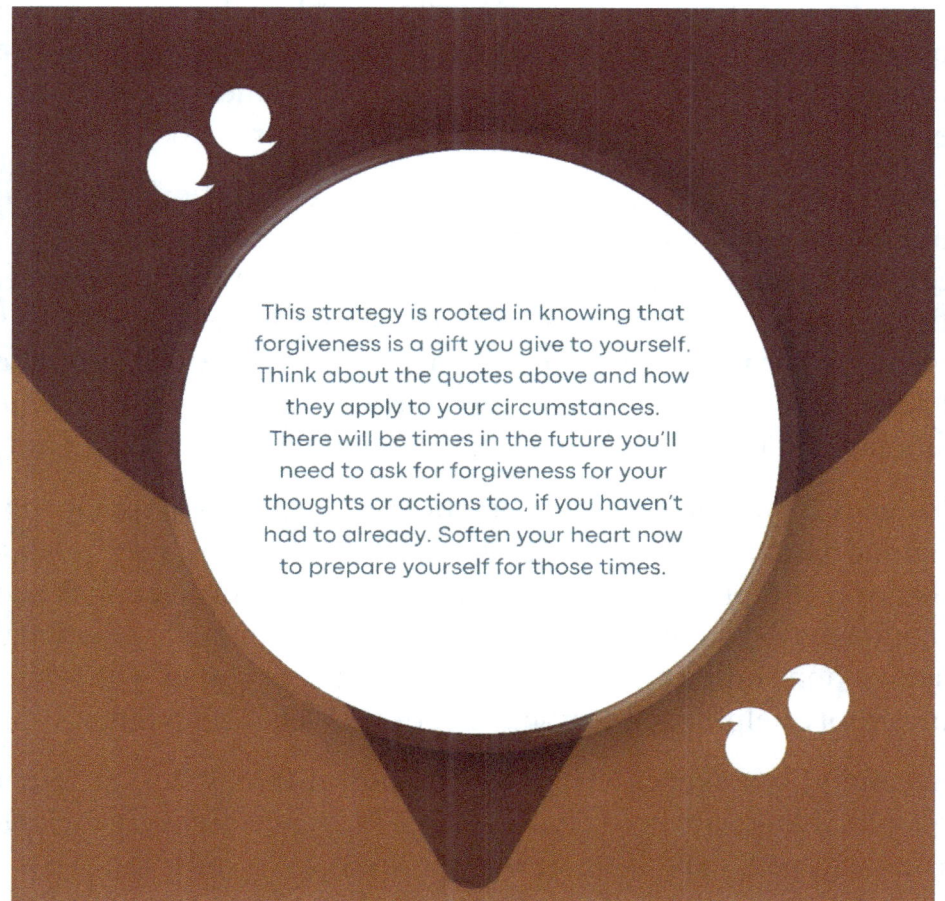

This strategy is rooted in knowing that forgiveness is a gift you give to yourself. Think about the quotes above and how they apply to your circumstances. There will be times in the future you'll need to ask for forgiveness for your thoughts or actions too, if you haven't had to already. Soften your heart now to prepare yourself for those times.

I want to point out three powerful truths about forgiveness that have helped me practice this critical discipline.

First of all, extending forgiveness is *not* the same as condoning behavior. That is a huge and important truth to keep in mind. And it's a crucial distinction during this time.

I struggled for so long (and periodically still do) trying to work out how to forgive. I worried that showing forgiveness would signal to my kids that I was okay with their dad's behavior. I sought counseling to discern what it would look like in my life. I prayed about being able to forgive as Jesus did, knowing that He forgave those who literally took His life. (And the betrayal I experienced, painful as it was, was nothing compared to *that*.)

My counselor shared a strategy with me that you may find helpful too. It's adapted from the teaching of Charles Stanley. She said to open a spreadsheet (I used an old-time spreadsheet from a pad I had lying around) and write out whatever I was having a hard time forgiving. Attach a price or cost to it in the "debit" column. Then, right below, add a "credit" for the same amount and physically cross out the amount owed, or the debt.

Whenever you feel resentment or unforgiveness popping up, remind yourself that you've already canceled that debt. Using that specific phrase makes the entire process transactional and minimizes the emotional aspect. For me, detaching the emotional connection from forgiveness—something I struggled with—was incredibly helpful as I learned to forgive such a deep hurt.

Secondly, forgiveness is going to look different for different people. If there are geographic miles of distance between you and your ex, you may have few opportunities to interact. To be honest, that may make forgiveness a little easier to extend at first.

(And as your life grows and your heart heals, it *does* get easier.) But if you live in the same city or town, you may need to be a bit more creative or proactive. Seek guidance from someone you trust as you navigate this step. Don't allow yourself to be guilted into any behavior or feeling. Remember, there is no guidebook that can tell you exactly what to do and how to move forward (including the book you're reading right now). This is a singular journey that you navigate on your own, at your own pace, and in your own way.

Remember, however, that boundaries do apply here. You must decide what you can and can't handle emotionally, and then establish your personal boundaries (see Chapter 5). For example, I have mixed feelings about meeting my ex's girlfriend, so for the time being, if she is at a family gathering, I may not attend. It's not out of vindictiveness; it's out of self-care. I'm not making a stink about it; I just won't be there. That may change down the road (boundaries sometimes do), but that's where I am right now.

Finally, forgiveness does not mean there are no consequences. Divorce breaks a relationship. It breaks it on a practical level, and it breaks it on a spiritual level. This is not something that can or should be brushed under the rug. Stashing a broken vase underneath a throw rug will only cause people to trip and possibly hurt themselves. Everyone can still see it, and most people will skirt around it.

But everyone knows something is there.

Other people will be hurt by your divorce. That's merely an observation, a statement of fact. It will affect your adult children; it may confuse and dismay your mutual friends. If your parents are still alive, it will most certainly hurt or at least affect them in some way. That's not to guilt trip you or make you feel worse than you may already be feeling. It's just to point out that you aren't the only one who will be dealing with forgiveness.

You are not alone.

YOUR TURN

You may not be ready to forgive, but you can start laying the groundwork now. Start praying for the ability to forgive, think about what forgiveness might look like, journal your thoughts, and (if you haven't started it already) engage in counseling. Do this as a gift to yourself.

PART 2
MOVING FORWARD WITH STRENGTH

10.
SUDDENLY SUPPORTING YOURSELF

"There are uses to adversity, and they don't reveal themselves until tested. Whether it's serious illness, (or) financial hardship ... difficulty can tap unexpected strengths."
~ Sonia Sotomayor

"If in trouble, focus on where you want to be rather than where you are!"
~ Somya Kedia

Note: Some topics not covered in the STRENGTHS framework are still important to address in a book about rebuilding your post-divorce life. In the next few chapters, I cover a few of these.

With divorce comes the reality of being financially self-supporting. And that means so much more than just paying the electric bill.

As I mentioned in the Introduction, many women in gray divorces were raised during a time when men took care of paying the bills, budgeting, and handling details pertaining to life and health insurance. I mean, it was as recently as 1974 when married women were first able to open a credit card without their husband's permission! Additionally, women like me may have chosen to stay home and take care of the children and all things domestic. While this is a bucket load of work in and of itself, it still leaves many of us vulnerable and to some extent ignorant of handling the whole financial picture.

Fortunately, we live in a day and age when spouses act as partners and both parties contribute to planning budgets and paying bills. But this responsibility can be overwhelming if we are suddenly responsible for that while also dealing with the emotional baggage of an impending divorce.

While men might not be used to handling the day-to-day finances, women are typically left with less to work with after a divorce at this age. Statistics bear witness to the fact that when couples face divorce after the age of fifty, the financial toll on women is much worse.[11]

I will never forget the first meeting I had with the financial planner I found after my divorce. I began by dispassionately describing my financial situation as best as I could. It was challenging, however, because when I looked at the numbers, I realized I was really behind the eight ball, so to speak.

Unfazed, he finally asked me a question that broke through my calm demeanor: "What do *you* want?" He asked it sincerely, to help us get started creating a plan that would move me forward financially. But it was at that point that I began to feel my financial knowledge was too sorely lacking, my vision too deeply blurred, and my goals and desires too muddled for my own good.

How would I ever be able to discern a clear and goal-driven way to get from "here" to "there," wherever "there" was?

Fortunately, my financial planner wasn't deterred by the tears that spilled over as we continued to explore the answers to his questions. And what began that afternoon in his office turned into something I'd never imagined.

I began to develop my financial literacy and discovered I actually enjoyed learning about money. Yep, me—the one who had always deferred to my ex and our (male) accountants, CPAs, and financial planners. The one who always claimed, "I don't have a head for numbers." The one who always thought she was much more of a wordsmith than a numbers person.

I began to study for licensing to become a certified financial planner. And my new-found mission became to help women who have been through a gray divorce take charge of their finances and create a solid financial future for themselves. If I can do it, anyone can!

Now, that doesn't mean you have to do what I did. But it could be that getting involved in community service, volunteer work, or learning more about a passion of yours will create an opportunity for a job or set you on a course of business ownership or entrepreneurship. I have often found that getting my eyes off *my* problems and exploring how I can help, serve, or support *others* comes back to me in spades.

There are no quick fixes here, but I want to encourage you to keep your head lifted. Stay expectant. Remain open. And don't be surprised when something comes your way to help you pay those bills—or even allow for a bit of extravagance in your life.

YOUR TURN

What steps do you need to take to get your finances in order? If making a list is too overwhelming, what's the *next* step you can take?

11.
DIVORCE AND YOUR ADULT CHILDREN

"How good and pleasant it is when brothers live together in unity."
~ Psalm 133:1

"Your feelings are valid and your voice matters."
~ Unknown

Wouldn't it be great if someone had the definitive answer for you about how to help your adult children through your divorce, a magic "relational pill" of sorts that would easily solve all possible scenarios?

In lieu of that, what I *can* offer you are some principles that worked for me, and others I uncovered in the research I dove into after my divorce. I'd suggest you do your own studying too. New strategies, discoveries, and research are constantly being developed that may offer you some creative ideas, hope, and help.

When a gray divorce happens to us, our children are most likely adults. But no matter their ages, your divorce also affects them. After all, the primary relationship they've known all their lives is about to become a thing of the past.

There's no predicting how it will affect them either. Personally, my kids have displayed various permutations of denial, anger, sadness, relief, and what seems like casual acceptance (all of which sound like the stages of grief to me).

Additionally, it may cause problems between or among siblings as they disagree with how others may be handling the situation. It may be especially difficult not to insert yourself into the argument, but work hard to fight that temptation. At this stage of their lives, their relationships are between each other. As important as it is not to have them choose between you and your ex-spouse, it's equally important that *you* don't choose sides in *their* disagreements.

Here are some questions I've found helpful to think about while navigating the effects of our divorce on our adult children:

How do I know if my adult children are hurting?

It's best to assume they are, even if (or because) they might not easily identify it. They might be extra supportive of you, or they may not talk to you about the divorce at all. They may cheer on your growth and personal development, or they may be dismissive or even resentful. They may be deep in denial and rationalize it by saying the divorce is between the two of you (which is true) and therefore doesn't impact their lives at all (which is not).

How can I help them through this?

Although your children are probably adults, you will always be their mother. And there's a certain amount of lifetime nurturing that goes along with that title.

- First and foremost, the best way to help them is to get counseling for *yourself*. Understandably, they may be the first people who try to help you through this difficult time, since they know both of you and may want to comfort one or both of you. But this inevitably puts them in the uncomfortable position of feeling like they have to take sides.

- Have the scary conversations with them. They're no doubt old enough to talk about their feelings, even if they're having a hard time processing them. The initial and early discussions are bound to be awkward and unsettling for both of you, and that's okay. If you need some good questions to get started, I've included a resource for useful journal prompts for adult children of divorce in the Recommended Resources section. The article titled "A Message from Your Adult Child About Your Divorce" also offers some terrific suggestions for conversation starters.

- Set healthy boundaries. Remember that boundaries are for *you*, not for them. All the concepts we talked about in Chapter 5 apply here, because your children are adults now too. Don't make them choose sides. Don't overshare. And just as important, be willing to accept *their* boundaries.

Just as you're not the only one working on forgiveness, you may find you and your adult kiddos have some intense emotions and feelings in common. Allow this painful time to foster mutual growth for and deepen the relationship between you.

YOUR TURN

If you have children, think about what issues have come up and how your relationship has been altered. While you (and they) are bound to make mistakes navigating this new terrain, keep short tabs on hurts and disagreements, and keep the channels of communication open. Use this page to make notes about what you plan to do to keep these relationships healthy and strong.

12.
ON BROKENNESS

"When you say, 'It's too hard now,' remember: It'll only be harder later. If it feels too hard, it'll only feel harder later. Choose your hard."
~ Unknown

"The biggest lesson I've learned is, 'It's okay.'... It's okay to be wrong. It's okay to get mad. It's okay to be flawed. It's okay to be happy. It's okay to move on."
~ Unknown

No matter who initiated your divorce, the net result is the same: a broken relationship. There may be more than one, actually, when you consider in-laws, confused friends, and hurt children. It's painful all around; there's no avoiding it.

Numerous analogies display how pain leads to growth. Seeds break ground as they reach through dirt to find the sun. Muscles break down during exercise as a person becomes stronger. Children experience "growing pains" as their young bodies develop. And, of course, there's the quintessential agony of childbirth that brings new life into the world.

These are all good visuals, but I believe the concept that brings the most hope, and in such a beautiful way, is the art of Kintsugi.

Kintsugi is an ancient Japanese art form where a piece of delicate pottery is broken and then put back together. What makes it special is that the ensuing cracks are *highlighted* with gold paint or gold leaf. They're not meant to be hidden or covered up. Instead, they are repaired in a way that draws attention to them, that emphasizes the damage while playing up the beauty that occurs as a result of the repair.

I think anyone who has gone through a divorce and is struggling to put their lives back together should have a piece of Kintsugi in their home. (And if you're looking for an encouraging gift for a divorced loved one, this is it!) While searching for one to purchase for myself, I came upon this thought shared by an artisan who goes by Wabi-Sabi Chic:

"Your scars and wounds ... are your beauty. Like broken objects mended with gold, we are all Kintsugi—the breakage and mending are all honest parts of our past and should be celebrated and not hidden. They are pieces and parts of who you are. Every beautiful thing is damaged. You're more beautiful for having been broken."[12]

I'm not saying we should celebrate divorce per se. As I explained in the introduction, I still believe in marriage for life. I take promises, commitments, and vows very seriously. But sometimes divorce happens. And when it happens to *you*, "you (can be) more beautiful for having been broken."

Why, I wonder, do we fear brokenness so much? When I stop to think about it, I realize that I'm not really afraid of dying. I just don't want it to hurt. If I had my choice, I'd prefer to pass on quietly and peacefully in my sleep. It's not the finality of it. It's the pain I want to avoid.

I don't think anyone *wants* to experience brokenness either. And in this season of life, I'm convinced what we, or I at least, truly fear isn't the breaking itself, but the pain that occurs during the process.

I remember the last time I gave birth, truly fearing the pain in a way I did not experience with my first four deliveries. I remember the handful of years I spent still married but painfully alone. I remember moving into my current home and all the "getting rid of" that had to occur as I downsized from a 2,800-square-foot, four-bedroom home with a two-car attached garage to a 1,300-square-foot townhouse. Crud, *that* was painful!

So how do we incorporate brokenness (and the pain that comes with it) into a beautiful, whole, and healthy life? Again, while there are some basic, tried-and-true principles, this looks different for everyone. Here's what worked for me:

- Feel the feels, but don't let them swallow you up. Get help and find support however you need it.

- Find ways to have fun. If you were married for a long time, this one may be challenging. You may be triggered by doing the fun things you'd done as a couple, which kind of defeats the purpose, doesn't it? So take some time to think about what you enjoyed *before* your marriage or some of the things you've done with girlfriends over the years. Better yet, do something totally different—something you've always wanted to do or to try and just never got around to.

- Be ready and eager to share the little victories you experience day to day, but don't go on and on about your pain with friends. While you may be doing it to be transparent, it can make other people uncomfortable. (Here's a little tip: If you can identify just *one* victory each day, you'll start to see more pop up over time.)

- Don't let yourself get stuck. When I was growing up, my stepmother used to remind me, "This too shall pass." I hated hearing it then, but the truth remains. If you need help finding ways to start moving on, discover some quick wins in Chapter 14.

- Buy yourself a piece of Kintsugi. Or, if you're feeling super-crafty, find an interesting or pretty piece of pottery and make one yourself. Placed in a prominent location, it will become a daily reminder of your beauty, strength, resilience, and ability.

We're all broken, dear friend. And then we move on.

YOUR TURN

Journal about your thoughts on brokenness. How does it manifest in your life? What affirmations might you need to start telling yourself to work toward healing and wholeness? Start putting together a way to Kintsugi your life.

13.
HOLIDAYS AND HAPPINESS

"The holiday season is a perfect time to reflect on our blessings and seek out ways to make life better for those around us."
~ Unknown

"Now is not the time to think of what you do not have. Think of what you can do with what there is."
~ Ernest Hemingway

Note: Many of the strategies outlined in this book will be helpful as you celebrate holidays after your divorce. If possible, read this chapter carefully and seek counseling (if necessary) <u>before</u> that first big occasion rolls around.

Post-divorce, long-held family traditions and expectations will be forever changed. Because of this, emotions, tempers, and feelings may run high and be volatile during these festive seasons. Along with other family members, you may feel like you're walking on eggshells. While that may be unavoidable soon after your divorce, it's never preferable—and it's rather difficult and unhealthy to maintain.

In other words, you may need to learn a new way to walk through the holidays. Here are some suggestions to help you get started.

You may discover you need to embrace simplicity in a new way. After my divorce, I moved into a much smaller townhouse and found it impractical to host big family gatherings like those I'd organized throughout my entire married life. My elder daughter and my eldest son's wife (my daughter-in-love), both of whom lived in spacious, party friendly homes, gladly took over the hosting role. I must admit, though, that it was hard for me to let go. And while I was happy they were willing to exercise hospitality, it took me a while to stop wishing *I* was still the "hostess with the mostest." With a smaller income, I also had to simplify gift giving (and stop comparing my gifts to those from others in the family). This is just a sampling of the opportunities you'll have to simplify the holidays you've celebrated over the years as a family. No doubt, others will present themselves, often when you least expect them. You'll do well to look at them as occasions for growth and creativity. Grieve the inevitable losses and changes, but as I've said before in this guide, don't get stuck there.

Through counseling, I discovered that part of taking care of myself was asking how *I* wanted to observe the holidays. What parties would I attend? How would I celebrate with the kids/grandkids and when? The Norman Rockwell Christmas—with the whole family gathered around a huge table groaning under the weight of a scrumptious meal and the lavishly decorated, ten-foot-tall tree in front of the fireplace with brightly wrapped presents nestled underneath—was a dream of the past. But with all those extras stripped away, I discovered a wonderful freedom. No more unreasonable expectations. No more (or at least, less) strain and stress. No more huge financial debt. I took the time to think about it in detail and decide what celebrating looked like *for me*.

However, this meant that I had to decide on my boundaries, and that wasn't something that could happen overnight. It was, and still is, a continual process of experimentation.

Remember, boundaries enable us to preserve our relationships. They allow us to behave authentically, in ways that align with our values. I discovered that knowing my boundaries also allowed me to be at peace with apparent contradictions. For example, I could forgive my ex while no longer trusting him. I could be curious about his life without condoning his behavior. And I could mourn and miss what might have been while living with joy in the present.

As a result, I gradually learned how to be gentle with myself. And as holidays come and go, I become a better student of my own preferences, abilities, limits of what I am able and willing to tolerate, and what truly brings me joy.

Think about it: *You* get to decide where and with whom you'd like to celebrate the holidays! The fact, for example, that I no longer have the "holidays central" home allows me to help my children move forward with establishing *their* family celebrations and be a part of those festivities. Because of this, I've developed a deep sense of gratitude. I get to watch them moving into their own adulthood and am part of the picture of what their families look like. What a privilege! Once I pivoted in my approach to celebrating the holidays, it opened a whole new world of blessings for which to be grateful.

Once again, let me point out the healing power of laughter. The holiday season can provide plenty of opportunities to deliver joy. Find the funny wherever and however you can. (And don't be afraid to laugh at yourself too!) Early on, your post-divorce sense of humor may come across to others as caustic or sarcastic, so you may need to keep your observations to yourself for a while. But as your heart heals and hope is renewed, your humor will naturally reflect and nurture the growing joy and optimism within you. Laugh deeply, Laugh often. And soon *you'll* be known as the person who lights up the room.

Finally, look for ways to help others during the holiday season. For years, I'd wanted to take our family to volunteer at a local soup kitchen for Thanksgiving. I know other families do this, but for various reasons, it didn't happen for us. To be clear, I'm not blaming anyone in my family for that. But my divorce stripped me of any excuses I'd made for not doing what my heart desired. As a reminder: The best way to heal and grow is to stop moping about our problems and find someone else to help. And while the power of laughter is healing, the power of service might be even more so. Just think about all the joy that could be unearthed when you draw on your sense of humor while you're serving others in the community. (Sounds like the best kind of "two-for" deal to me!)

YOUR TURN

How will holidays with your family look different as you create your new life? How would you like to celebrate them? What boundaries will you have to set? Make some notes here. After you've pondered your preferences, set aside some casual time to talk with your adult children and come up with a plan together.

14.
QUICK WINS

"May you be strengthened by yesterday's rain, walk straight in tomorrow's wind, and cherish each moment of the sun today."
~ Ojibwe Saying

"Over the short term, we regret action over inaction. Over the long term, it's the opposite."
~ Daniel Pink

A study I came across recently revealed that, as people age, they were more affected by regretting what they *didn't* do, as opposed to regretting actions that may have been deemed mistakes[13]. Considering the season in which I'm writing this book, that totally makes sense. I'm finding I can live with short-term regrets about awkward moments, relational faux pas, or saying the wrong thing at the wrong time. But I don't want to waste my energy regretting those "coulda, shoulda, woulda" moments. It took me a long time to get where I am, after all. I want to enjoy whatever time I have left.

So in this last section, I want to share some (relatively) quick wins you can use to start moving forward. These, too, don't fit in neatly with the STRENGTHS concepts, but they've often helped me in a pinch. As always, use the journaling page at the end of this chapter to make your own notes or tweak something you read here.

Find support. This will look different for everyone, but we all need help. Healing from a divorce and creating what amounts to a brand new life is no time for pride. Get counseling, even if it's only for a short while, and then consider life coaching or some way to start reframing your mindset and developing a more positive approach to life. Look for mentors and seek training when you need it, especially if you're also embarking on a new career or trying to get back into something you did years ago. I'd also suggest looking for a good financial advisor. Understand that *you* are now responsible for providing for your old age. Don't be scared by this, but *do* find someone you trust who can help you prepare for those years.

Think about important questions and journal your answers. Remember the question my new financial advisor (of all people) asked me that afternoon in his office: "What do *you* want to do?" It seemed like an odd query until he explained the motivation for it. Money is simply a tool and should be used as such. As with any tool, you need to know what you're trying to accomplish so you use the correct tool *and* use it appropriately. Surprisingly (to me, at least), I couldn't answer his question right away. But it *did* inspire me to start thinking about it, along with other questions:

Do I have the right people around me to ask for help?

What has been true for me my whole life that doesn't have to be true for the rest of my life? Stated differently, what can I leave behind? What do I *need* to leave behind?

Am I interruptible? Interruptions often open the door to opportunities. Who or what does God keep putting in my path?

Whatever's been given to me was not meant to stay with me. What has been given to me that I need to give away?

While these questions aren't necessarily connected, I found that once I started thinking deeper thoughts, deeper questions arose. And the answers enriched my life.

Look up. A friend of mine who is also a mental health therapist once ran this exercise in a group we were in. She told us to lift our faces up and look at the ceiling (you can also do this outside and look at the clouds). Keeping your face uplifted, move your eyes down and look at the ground. (No cheating, now—keep your face up!) How far do you get? Next, turn your face down and move your eyes so that you're looking up at the ceiling or sky. How successful are you? Either way, you'll note that no matter which direction your head is pointed, your eyes follow. It is *impossible* to see the ground when your head is facing the sky, and vice versa.

Go ahead and make the connection to your life. If you're having a difficult day, go outside, sit in a chair or on the steps, and look up! If you can't get dressed, do it in your jammies. The point is: start training your body to look up, and your mind is sure to follow. As a favorite Bible verse of mine puts it, "I lift up my eyes to the mountains—where does my help come from? My help comes from the LORD, the Maker of heaven and earth."[14]

Do a physical chore. I have two go-to tasks: clean up the kitchen or hand-wash the car. I'll admit that the car gets washed far less than the kitchen gets cleaned, but that's not the point. This might sound simplistic, but it's really not. When we immerse ourselves in a project that involves our minds *and* bodies, something magical happens. I'm sure there is a scientific explanation for it, but since I'm not a scientist, you'll have to settle with my first-person experience. Maybe it has something to do with focusing on something not related to our problem/pain/issue, maybe it's the sense of satisfaction you get when it's done, or maybe it's the physical tiredness you feel that was truly earned. Whatever the case, do the go-to chore that feels best to you and pay attention to how you feel when you're done. It hasn't solved everything, of course, but you may find you've gained a new sense of momentum. And at this stage of the game, we need to celebrate even the little wins.

Turn on some tunes. My college degree (oh-so-many years ago) is in music therapy. Even "way back then," I learned about the transformative power of music. And yes, Virginia, there *is* science and research behind this concept. In regards to emotional healing, "Music therapy has shown promise in providing a safe and supportive environment for healing trauma and building resilience while decreasing anxiety levels and improving the functioning of depressed individuals."[15] In less academic terms, who doesn't love a good tune? I have an entire playlist of songs to get me started in the morning, and another for when I need to feel stronger and focus on being an overcomer. Personally, I'm a fan of music from the seventies and eighties, and there is a treasure trove of helpful tunes available. (See the Recommended Resources page for information about my "Silver Grooves" playlist.)

Maintain hope. While I'm not a sports fan, I have sat through my fair share of Super Bowls, car races, and soccer games. I've seen enough comebacks, upsets, and successful Hail Mary passes to understand that you can't always be sure of the score before the second half of the game is played. In other words: it ain't over 'till it's over. That, to me, is the essence of hope. Despite what has gone before, it's always possible for the future to be better.

Practice living with hope. Yes, it *does* take practice.

Be generous. Seth Godin once said, "The path forward is about curiosity, generosity, and connection."[16] Although he was referring to creative work, I believe this quote can also be applied to our lives in general. Post-divorce, I began to look at my life like that: as a piece of art that I had the responsibility, privilege, and joy of creating. Generosity included making financial donations, but it also included sharing my time and abilities. Looking outside of myself and my problems to see how I could help and contribute to others' success and joy was immensely helpful. Although this wasn't my intent, developing the gift of generosity became one of those things that seemed to bless me more than those I was attempting to bless. I challenge and encourage you to try it too.

Help someone else. This is related to being generous, but I'm specifically referring to helping someone who is also going through a divorce. If you're early in the process yourself, you might want to wait on this. As you proceed, however, you'll be learning and growing in myriad ways, and it's amazing how often you'll come across people who could benefit from hearing a word of encouragement or inspiration from your story.

Don't overthink or overdo it, however. Offer a listening ear without giving advice. Sit and grieve with them in silence or tears. Take them out for ice cream to give them a change of scenery. Keeping it simple is wise and almost always appreciated. When I need a reminder about this, I turn to a children's book called *And Rabbit Listened*, the tender story of how a sad young boy is finally comforted by a quiet rabbit after all the other animals try to make him feel better by telling him what to do.

Write your epitaph. No, I'm not being morbid—hear me out! Too often, people on their deathbeds are consumed with regrets, wishing they could get a mulligan, a do-over, another chance to do things differently. Try this: Take time to write six or so words or phrases you want others to use about you when you die. If you're really getting into it, go ahead and write more. The point is to describe yourself as the person you want to be so that you can start living it out *now*. What a gift you're giving to yourself! You don't have to be going through a divorce to try this activity, of course. But since you're here, creating a brand-new future for yourself, why not be intentional about it?

Assess your choices. We all have choices. Period. Full stop. Now, we may not *like* the choices we have. We may feel as if we're in between a rock and a hard place. And we may not always be able to see our options. (If the latter is the case for you, do the following activity with someone you trust and who knows you well.) Here's what I want you to do. Grab pen and paper and start writing. Make a list of the choices you are facing right now. Underneath each one, make a pro and con list of your possible decisions. I guess it's not really fair to call this one a "quick" win. Done well, it could take a few days or more. As you start to get these choices out of your head and onto paper, you'll realize a few things. One is that you may not have as many decisions to make as you think. And the ones you do have may not really be urgent ones, which means you can stress less and breathe easier. Finally, seeing the options you have may prove to be incredibly empowering.

Get to know yourself better. It was a bit embarrassing to realize that, as a sixty-year-old woman, I had trouble answering when my financial advisor asked me what I wanted to do. Later, a business coach (again, of all people) challenged me with this activity. She told me to make a list of twenty things I want to *do*, twenty things I want to *have*, twenty things I *love to do*, and the accomplishments I am most proud of in my life. Whew—talk about getting to know yourself better! Those are lists that, even today, are still open ended and to which I add something quite often. Or remove something. They're living and changing, much as I am, and reflect the person I believe I am today and want to become tomorrow.

This next strategy is one I learned from entrepreneur and business coach Amy Porterfield. Ask people to share what they think you're about. Explain to them that you're researching yourself and need their honest feedback. If you're already in business, make the request related to your field. Or make it a personal request, and ask people what character traits come to mind when they think of you. (Be aware that this activity can put you in a tremendously vulnerable spot. While the comments you'll receive will most likely be positive and encouraging, make sure you're in a space where you can handle feedback.)

A final step as you get to know yourself is to create a personal self-care checklist. Write a list of ten things you want to improve in this healing season of your life. On a scale of one to ten, rate yourself on them now. Some of the items I wrote down were:

1. Do I connect with myself daily (emotions and physical health)?

2. How compassionate am I being with myself?

3. How often do I pray?

4. Do I express gratitude daily?

5. Am I doing something to improve my quality of life (learning, reading, etc.)?

Tuck the list away after you grade it, and pull it out again in a few weeks or months for review. Regrade it, tuck it away and review it again a few months after *that*. Each time you review it, celebrate the success you've achieved.

Because there *will* be successes as you move ahead. I promise.

Slow down. I've said this before, but it bears repeating: Post-divorce growth and recovery is not a race. *Please* don't try to rush it! And don't compare your life or adjustment with anyone else's. I was strongly reminded of this a while back while listening to a sermon about Martha and Mary, in Luke 10. For those of you unfamiliar with the story, one evening, sisters Mary and Martha were enjoying a visit from their friend Jesus, at home. Well, Mary was, at least. Martha was busy with the hustle and bustle that often comes with hosting guests: preparing and serving the meal, attending to people's needs, etc. To her, it appeared Mary was totally "checked out." She offered Martha no help, which increasingly frustrated her sister, who finally had enough. Martha complained bitterly to Jesus and asked Him to encourage Mary to help her. Jesus's response was surprising (and I admit, if I were Martha, I would have found it a tad offensive too). "Martha, Martha, you are worried and upset about many things, but only one thing is needed. Mary has chosen what is better, and it will not be taken away from her."[17]

Jesus was pointing out that wherever we focus our attention gets our affection. Rushing around and worrying about the details is a distraction from what truly matters. You and I need to be much more like Mary than Martha. Prioritizing everyone else's needs over the years was part of the reason I got here in the first place. Constant hustle and bustle without settling in and enjoying the present inevitably leads to burnout and bitterness, and who wants to be around anyone with those traits?

I needed to be with people, and I needed the support and love from those who cared about me. But I also needed to learn to chill. More importantly, I needed to seek comfort and rest, in order to experience the renewal that rest provides.

YOUR TURN

Which one (or two) of the quick wins listed here are you going to try first? Or, do you have another one? Write it down to be accountable to yourself. Or better yet, a friend.

15.
FINAL THOUGHTS

"When you come out of the storm, you won't be the same person who walked in. That's what the storm is all about."
~ *Haruki Murakami*

"You may encounter many defeats, but you must not be defeated. In fact, it may be necessary to encounter the defeats so you can know who you are, what you can rise from, how you can still come out of it." ~ *Maya Angelou*

If you've gotten this far in this book, congratulations!

If you're reading this for a loved one, you have the truest heart of a friend. I trust that whoever you are supporting through this difficult season will feel blessed by your care and concern.

If you're reading this for yourself—if you've struggled or are struggling to regain your footing during this painful life transition, yet you're reaching for help and support in different ways—kudos to you, friend. This is part of the process, and it means you're on your way.

But the journey never ends.

Even if you someday remarry (which should not necessarily be anyone's ultimate goal) and live happily ever after, you do so as a changed person. Not damaged, mind you, but most certainly changed.

Time alone heals nothing, but time plus an intentional approach to healing and self-improvement works wonders. Yes, there are days when I still feel the bitter sting of betrayal from someone I once loved. But then there are those other days—many more of them as time moves on—when I look back and see how I've grown. I look back and see how what I once considered to be the end of the world was merely life-altering.

What Satan had intended for evil, God redeemed in His grace.

I am forever changed, and I am eternally grateful.

16.
Recommended Resources

Books:

- Everything is Figureoutable by Marie Forleo
- Keep Moving: Notes on Loss, Creativity and Change. Maggie Smith
- What Happened to You? Conversations on Trauma, Resilience, and Healing, Bruce D. Perry and Oprah Winfrey
- Empty Nest Awakening: Weaving the Threads of Your Passions into Purpose by Ruthie Gray
- The Broken Way: A Daring Path into the Abundant Life by Ann Voskamp
- Boundaries: When to Say Yes, How to Say No To Take Control of Your Life, Dr. Henry Cloud and Dr. John Townsend
- The Practice: Shipping Creative Work by Seth Godin
- Your Post-Divorce Compass: Practical Real-World Advice for the Newly Single, Michael R. Dunham
- Curtains Wide Open: Anthology of Insights for the Women We Were compiled by Melissa Trumble and Leslie Lindsey Davis

- Home Will Never Be The Same Again: A Guide for Adult Children of Grey Divorce by Carol R. Hughes and Bruce R. Fredenberg

For more blog posts, articles, studies, journal prompts, and other resources, explore patfenner.me/gray-resources

17.
NOTES

¹Greg Iacurci, "'Gray Divorce' Has Doubled since the '90s—and the Financial Risk Is High for Women," CNBC, March 23, 2024, https://www.cnbc.com/2024/03/23/why-gray-divorce-is-a-significant-financial-risk-for-women.html.

²Kendra Cherry, "Why So Many Older Couples Are Falling Victim to the Gray Divorce Phenomenon," Verywell Mind, Updated September 24, 2024, https://www.verywellmind.com/gray-divorce-8646068; "What's Behind the Grey Divorce Revolution?" High Swartz Law Firm, April 18, 2024, https://highswartz.com/legal-insights/family-law/grey-divorce-revolution/.

³Daniel de Visé, "More Americans are Splitting After 50. Financial Planning Tips for a 'Gray Divorce,'" *USA Today*, January 28, 2024, https://www.usatoday.com/story/money/2024/01/28/gray-divorce-more-americans-split-after-50/72337078007/.

⁴Melissa Trumble, Leslie Lindsey Davis, Jenny Baltazar, Jennifer Bloome, Helen Edwards, Audrey Faust, Pat Fenner, Carole Filion, Pam Karlen, Lindsey Maria, and Romine Lee Ann, *Curtains Wide Open: Anthology of Insights for the Women We Were* (published by the authors, 2023), Chapter 5.

⁵"Trust," *Psychology Today,* https://bit.ly/4cqMWgh.

⁶Prov. 4:27

[7]Emily H. Sanders, LMFT (@Emily.sanders.therapy), "Going to therapy is a gift to yourself." Instagram, June 18, 2024, https://bit.ly/3BYnamn

[8]"Superblooms in California," Theodore Payne Foundation," https://theodorepayne.org/superbloom/.

[9]Sahil Bloom, "The Parable of the Farmer & the Horse," *The Curiosity Chronicle*, https://www.sahilbloom.com/newsletter/the-parable-of-the-farmer-the-horse.

[10]Shana Schutte, "Even Jesus Had Boundaries," Wisdom Hunters, May 2, 2023, https://www.wisdomhunters.com/even-jesus-had-boundaries/.

[11]Mary Payne Bennett and Cecile Lengacher, "Humor and Laughter May Influence Health: III. Laughter and Health Outcomes," Wiley Onlinbe Library, https://doi.org/10.1093/ecam/nem041.

[12]"We Are All Imperfect. Celebrate Your Unique Beauty," Wabi-Sabi Chic's official website, https://www.wabisabichic.com/wabi-sabi-shibui.html.

[13]Daniel Pink, "How to Understand Regret—and 2 Ways to Avoid It," Daniel H. Pink's official website, August 22, 2011, https://www.danpink.com/2011/08/how-to-understand-regret-and-2-ways-to-avoid-it/.

[14]Ps. 121:1-2

[15]Sonja Aalbers, Laura Fusar-Poli, Ruth E. Freeman, Marinus Spreen, Johannes C.F. Ket, Annemiek C. Vink, Anna Maratos, Mike Crawford, Xi-Jing Chen, and Christian Gold, "Music

Therapy for Depression," Cochrane Database of Systematic Reviews, November 16, 2017, https://doi.org/10.1002/14651858.cd004517.pub3.

[16]Seth Godin, quote from the *Practice: Shipping Creative Work*, Goodreads.com, https://www.goodreads.com/quotes/10882725-the-path-forward-is-about-curiosity-generosity-and-connection-these.

[17]Luke 10:38-42

www.ingramcontent.com/pod-product-compliance
Lightning Source LLC
Chambersburg PA
CBHW070435010526
44118CB00014B/2053